BRAIN DAMAGE AND
MENTAL RETARDATION

Second Edition

BRAIN DAMAGE AND MENTAL RETARDATION

A Psychological Evaluation

Edited by

J. L. KHANNA, Ph.D.

Associate Professor, Department of Psychiatry
University of Tennessee College of Medicine
Memphis, Tennessee

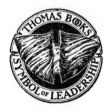

CHARLES C THOMAS · PUBLISHER
Springfield · Illinois · U.S.A.

Published and Distributed Throughout the World by

CHARLES C THOMAS • PUBLISHER

BANNERSTONE HOUSE

301-327 East Lawrence Avenue, Springfield, Illinois, U.S.A.

With THOMAS BOOKS *careful attention is given to all details of manufacturing and design. It is the Publisher's desire to present books that are satisfactory as to their physical qualities and artistic possibilities and appropriate for their particular use.* THOMAS BOOKS *will be true to those laws of quality that assure a good name and good will.*

Printed in the United States of America

W-2

CONTRIBUTORS

A. BARCLAY, PH.D., *Associate Professor, Department of Psychology; Director, Developmental Psychology Program, Saint Louis, University, Saint Louis, Missouri*

JERRY N. BOONE, PH.D., *Training Coordinator, Child Development Center, The University of Tennessee College of Medicine, Memphis, Tennessee*[1]

CONRAD CONSALVI, PH.D., *Assistant Professor, Department of Psychology, Memphis State University, Memphis, Tennessee*[2]

CHARLES P. DEMINICO, M.D., *Assistant Professor, Department of Psychiatry, The University of Tennessee College of Medicine, Memphis, Tennessee*[3]

MARY I. DUWALL, PH.D., *Assistant Professor and Clinical Psychologist, University of Alabama Medical Center, Birmingham, Alabama*

SUSAN W. GRAY, PH.D., *Professor, George Peabody College for Teachers, Nashville, Tennessee*

F. S. HILL, M.D., *Associate Clinical Professor of Pediatrics, The University of Tennessee College of Medicine, Memphis, Tennessee*

T. S. HILL, M.D., *Director, Brain Research Institute; Professor of Psychiatry, The University of Tennessee College of Medicine, Memphis, Tennessee*

J. T. JABBOUR, M.D., *Pediatric Neurologist, Child Development Center, The University of Tennessee College of Medicine, Memphis, Tennessee*

WALLACE A. KENNEDY, PH.D., *Staff Chairman, Human Development Clinic, Florida State University, Tallahassee, Florida*

PRABHA KHANNA, PH.D., *Assistant Professor of Psychiatry and Clinical Psychology, Division of Psychology, The University of Tennessee College of Medicine, Memphis, Tennessee*

LEON LEBOVITZ, PH.D., *School Psychologist, Division of Guidance,*

---

[1]*Now Professor, Department of Psychology, Memphis State University, Memphis, Tennessee.*

[2]*Now Associate Professor, Department of Psychology, American University, Beirut, Lebanon.*

[3]*Now Associate Professor, Department of Psychiatry, J. H. Miller Mental Health Center, University of Florida, Gainesville, Florida.*

Testing and Pupil Adjustment, Board of Education, Memphis, Tennessee

HENRY LELAND, PH.D., *Director of Psychology, The Ohio State University, Mental Retardation Program, Columbus, Ohio*

RAY W. MACKEY, M.D., *Associate Professor of Pediatric Neurology, The University of Tennessee College of Medicine, Memphis, Tennessee*

W. THEODORE MAY, PH.D., *Associate Professor of Psychiatry and Clinical Psychology, Division of Psychology, The University of Tennessee College of Medicine, Memphis, Tennessee*

MARTIN A. MENDELSON, PH.D., *Acting Head, Section on Behavioral Sciences, Perinatal Research Branch, National Institute of Neurological Diseases and Blindness, National Institutes of Health, Bethesda, Maryland*

GERALD R. PASCAL, PH.D., *Research Professor of Psychiatry, Department of Psychiatry, University of Mississippi Medical Center, Jackson, Mississippi*

WENTWORTH QUAST, PH.D., *Associate Professor, Division of Clinical Psychology, Departments of Psychiatry and Neurology, Pediatrics, and Psychology, University of Minnesota Medical Center, Minneapolis, Minnesota*

RALPH M. REITAN, PH.D., *Professor of Psychology (Neurology); Director, Neuropsychology Laboratory, Indiana University Medical Center, Indianapolis, Indiana*

ALAN O. ROSS, PH.D., *Chief Psychologist, Pittsburgh Child Guidance Center, Pittsburgh, Pennsylvania*

HERBERT W. SMITH, PH.D., *Associate Director, University of Tennessee Medical Units Computer Center; Assistant Professor, Psychiatry and Clinical Psychology, The University of Tennessee College of Medicine, Memphis, Tennessee*

ROBERT ALLEN UTTERBACK, M.D., *Professor and Chairman, Division of Neurology, The University of Tennessee College of Medicine, Memphis, Tennessee*

WILLIAM J. VON LACKUM, PH.D., *Professor and Chairman, Division of Psychology, The University of Tennessee College of Medicine, Memphis, Tennessee*

PREFACE TO THE FIRST EDITION

IN THE RECENT PAST there has been an increasing concern about the area of mental retardation, particularly with reference to brain damage. An assessment of the current status of our knowledge in this area and the delineation of new and, hopefully, fruitful lines of inquiry would be of considerable value both to investigators and practitioners.

Keeping this goal in mind, the Division of Psychology and the Department of Psychiatry of the University of Tennessee College of Medicine decided to hold an institute on this topic, and sought financial support for this purpose from the Division of Chronic Diseases of the United States Public Health Service. The present volume is an outgrowth of this institute,[1] held at the University of Tennessee College of Medicine on February 23, 24 and 25, 1966.

The planners of this institute felt that problems in the area of mental retardation and brain damage were not the province of any single discipline; that effective consideration required both intra- and interdisciplinary exchanges of ideas. Contributors and discussants were therefore selected from experimental, clinical, social and developmental psychology, as well as psychiatry, neurology and pediatric neurology.

In preparing the manuscript, it was decided to summarize the discussants' remarks instead of presenting them verbatim. While summarizing, the editor sought to reflect faithfully the content and tone of the presentation.

Although primary responsibility for the organization of the institute was undertaken by the undersigned, frequent advice and help was sought from members of the faculty of the University of Tennessee's Division of Psychology and Department of Psychiatry. Dr. Nelms B. Boone, Regional Mental Retardation Consultant (Region IV) of the Department of

---

[1]This institute was supported by the PHS Grant No. MR4504A66(T).

vii

Health, Education, and Welfare, gave valuable suggestions for the organization of the institute. Mrs. Joanne Lippy and Mrs. Rosalind Griffin, Division of Psychology, University of Tennessee College of Medicine, undertook the difficult task of typing the manuscript.

Thanks are due to all of the foregoing organizations and individuals for making possible both the institute and this book.

J. L. KHANNA, PH.D.

PREFACE TO THE SECOND EDITION

T HE FIRST EDITION of the book has been well received, and it was decided to publish a Second Edition in view of the continued demand.

All the principal contributors were contacted before the preparation of the manuscript for the Second Edition. Dr. Wallace A. Kennedy and Dr. Henry Leland have revised and brought up-to-date the chapters on "Poverty and the Brain" and on "An Overview of the Problem of the Psychological Evaluation in Mental Retardation." These chapters were rewritten by the authors so that the discussants' comments are still quite pertinent.

J. L. KHANNA, PH.D.

CONTENTS

BRAIN DAMAGE AND
MENTAL RETARDATION

I

AN OVERVIEW OF THE PROBLEM OF THE PSYCHOLOGICAL EVALUATION IN MENTAL RETARDATION

Henry Leland, Ph.D.

In February, 1963, President Kennedy presented to the Congress of the United States a historic message on mental illness and mental retardation. Today we have an opportunity to examine the field and to review the progress that this nation has made in some of the areas of mental retardation since President Kennedy's message.

Obviously, we are not endowed with the sources of information and resources which would make a complete overview of progress possible. But we can look at some of the things which the President's Panel on Mental Retardation outlined, as well as some of the more obvious areas of progress which have evolved. We will approach this question from three general aspects:

First, a discussion of the types of individuals to whom we are referring when we speak of evaluating the mentally retarded. Who, in the United States, are the individuals with whom we must be involved and what portion of the total problem is represented by our particular efforts?

Second, we will look at the developing treatment and rehabilitation services and facilities. If we are going to discuss the problem of the evaluation of the mentally retarded, we must also consider the consumer. For whom are we evaluating individuals and for what purpose are we making this evaluation?

Third, we will consider the function of evaluations in terms of the relative relationships between a system of classification on one hand and a diagnostic process on the other.

We might, for a moment, recall some of the things President

3

Kennedy (1963) described to Congress. For example, he indicated that mental retardation ranks as a major national health, social and economic problem:

> It disables ten times as many people as diabetes, twenty times as many as tuberculosis, twenty-five times as many as muscular dystrophy, and 600 times as many as infantile paralysis. About 400,000 children are so retarded they require constant care or supervision. More than 200,000 of these are in residential institutions. There are between five and six million mentally retarded children and adults—an estimated 3 percent of the population. Yet, despite these statistics and despite an admirable effort by private voluntary associations, until a decade ago, not a single state health department offered any special community services for the mentally retarded or their families.

Now we find that, in some respects, the picture has become worse. Improved case-finding techniques are beginning to show that the accepted figure of 3 per cent is probably too low if we consider all who function at a retarded level. We have the variable statistic, for example, from the Onondaga Study in 1953 (New York State, 1955) which indicated 2 per cent was probably a fair figure for preschool age, 3 per cent was probably a fair figure for postschool age, but that 10 per cent was probably a closer figure for the school age itself. Now, of course, there is no pretense that the child becomes retarded by going to school nor that he becomes cured by leaving school. (Rather, these statistics seem to indicate that the national figure of 3 per cent is probably representative of numbers with which most of us as professionals in the field will be involved. Nonetheless, there is also a large backlog of functionally retarded individuals whom we may not see under that label. They will probably emerge as part of a social problem through other areas of public concern such as welfare or unemployment—marginal individuals who have employment during periods of prosperity but who lose their employment during periods of want.) We may also raise the question of the large number of individuals still within the employable age who, because of technological unemployment, are without jobs and because of their marginal level of retardation, are unable to benefit from standard retraining efforts. This group of individuals as borderline or marginal retardates swells the problem with which we are dealing beyond the 3 per cent originally indicated.

This raises a number of very important questions in the matter of evaluation, particularly as they relate to sensory impairment, questions of brain damage, questions of cultural deprivation, and interrelated factors involving both brain damage, and cultural deprivation and their interaction. Furthermore, we have to recognize that when we look at the area of cultural deprivation a rather interesting phenomenon seems to develop. Generally speaking, there are no major social problems in the area of mental health or physical health which are most predominant in the low socioeconomic groups. Thus, cultural deprivation makes an individual a high risk for mental retardation, schizophrenia, alcoholism, narcotic addiction, divorce, tuberculosis, etc. Now, if poor socioeconomic conditions make the individual a high risk for all of these kinds of problems, then the socioeconomic conditions per se would not seem to be specific for any one of them; therefore, we are really dealing with a vast group of interrelationships. This does not in any way deny the role of deprivation in the development of retardation but does underline the fact that many other factors of human development must be considered. For example, the papers which Stein and Susser (1960) presented at the *London Conference on Mental Retardation* indicate that the particular label the individual received was every bit as much dependent on his socioeconomic origins as on any other one factor. They also indicated that, moving up the socioeconomic ladder, the same individual with the same behavioral characteristics would be diagnosed in a different way as a means of avoiding possible social stigma or definitive types of labels which might make the individual less of a rehabilitation candidate or less socially acceptable. These things being considered, we must suggest that the people we will be evaluating will be those who, for one reason or another, have not been able to cope with their environment. The American Association on Mental Deficiency has described this specific factor as *adaptive behavior*. The AAMD definition on mental retardation states: "Mental retardation refers to a subaverage general intellectual functioning which originates during the developmental period and is associated with impairment in adaptive behavior" (AAMD, 1961). This definition includes the subaverage intellectual functioning which the Onondaga Study emphasized. It includes elements which later speakers will discuss in reference to the developmental period. It also recognizes the relationship between cultural deprivation (as one of the sources of "subaverage general intellectual functioning") and the developmental period. But, let us also emphasize that the individual is still not really being labeled as mentally retarded unless there is also an impairment in adaptive behavior, or, in other words, unless there is also an inability to cope with the surrounding environment in terms of the requirements of that environment.

Therefore, the real answer to my original question of why studies are able to find 10 per cent of the school-age group and only 3 per cent of a postschool-age group retarded is because the missing per cent did not demonstrate impairments in adaptive behavior at that time. They were able, somehow or other, to become absorbed into the community and, to gain invisibility. Now we are getting new information indicating that their level of coping is not entirely what we would wish it to be, but that they are able to cope to the extent that there is no longer any need for the retarded label. So, for the purposes of this conference on evaluation, we are speaking primarily of that group of mentally retarded individuals who have not been able to cope. This group requires help and support through public clinics, special education classes, vocational rehabilitation services, geriatric services, etc., because the retardation is interfering with the ability to function in society. This requires further research, and much of this research is presently going forward.

The second question asked why we are making these evaluations. We have to consider the major aspect of President Kennedy's message. Both the message and the specific legislation which grew out of it were based on a proposed expansion in community programming and community services. Certainly the legislation which has grown out of this, the expansion both of community mental health and community mental retardation services, the increased legislation for comprehensive programs, the legislation providing for university-affiliated community services, etc., are indications of the type of consideration being given to this way of dealing with the problem. What has occurred is an expansion of all types of community services in the areas of both public health and mental health. The present programs in the War on Poverty, particularly those aspects of the program involving such things as Operation Head Start, are a continuation of this effort. This is not a question of case-finding. It is hoped all disadvantaged individuals in the community will receive the benefits of these programs whether they had previously decided they were mentally retarded or brain damaged. The preventive qualities of Head Start, or the preventive qualities of any kind of preschool programming aimed at developing the ability to cognize and learn in the culturally deprived child, will effectively help him to avoid developing into a mentally retarded child; thus it will reduce the load on our special education programs. In fact, if this preschool program could be carried out as we envision it, the need for EMR programs would be reduced. We could put the emphasis where it really belongs, on the trainable youngster whose needs are as related to medical and psychological factors as they are to deprivation. Again, we consider these medical and psychological problems to be an outgrowth of the disadvantaged background, so correction of the poverty problem will also help reduce these allied difficulties.

We need to consider the development of three essential service levels of treatment, training and rehabilitation. The first is represented by the local facilities, the special education classes, public health nurses, remedial teachers, local physicians, school psychologists, counselors, and others who come into contact, at the community level, with retarded individuals. It must be emphasized that these are not local facilities as they might appear in New York City, Chicago or Memphis, but are rather local facilities as they might appear in some of the small five to ten thousand population communities which dot our nation, where it is probable that there would not be more than one or two such individuals available. In other words, where a group of nonexperts will be dealing with retardation at its source, at the point where, if something effective could be done, *the more serious aspects of retardation might not have to develop.* This is the heart blood of the whole question because, if the retardation can be modified at the local level (and particularly during the preschool ages), it will not be necessary to talk of additional beds in state schools or hospitals. There would be no need to talk of the expansion of residential institutions but, instead as has occurred in adult psychiatry, of the reduction of beds and the changing of these services to fit the actual needs of the community. So we need to consider first, at this local level, those types of evaluations which may be conducted by a school psychologist or may be the findings of a teacher or public health nurse. The child will receive certain kinds of services as a result of the minimal sort of evaluation; therefore, materials are needed which will provide this local service with information from which it can derive guidelines to provide appropriate service. I do not want to minimize the importance of this type of local service. It is here that we find the special programs, the sheltered workshops, and the other programs of this sort; therefore, it is at the local level that a vast amount of education must go forward. Evaluation techniques must be developed which will aid this kind of programming so that nurses, physicians and others will have a more realistic understanding of our goals at this level. However, it is also at this level where most of the errors in labeling are made. These errors occur most often in relation to the disadvantaged and to national minorities. Therefore, these evaluation techniques must be based on the actual behaviors of the child rather than on the abstract, sometimes irrelevant concepts, such as IQ. What will be accomplished here is an application of the treatment and training programs in mental retardation which have been tried and tested, and which concern those aspects of the problem for which we think we have a known answer. We cannot expect much beyond this, but if this is accomplished in a systematic and carefully organized manner, we would be far ahead of our present status.

The next level is that of the comprehensive centers (the language of enabling legislation). These we usually develop on a regional or "zonal" basis and thus maintain some of the advantages of local contact. This level needs to be considered in two lights. The first, and perhaps the most important, is that we should not begin talking about mental health centers and mental retardation centers as though they were two separate and distinct things. It would be disastrous to begin talking about separate mental health and retardation centers at the local level because the possibility of manning such centers would be almost nil. Where we have one, possibly two, school psychologists in a system, we certainly cannot expect one to be dealing only with mental health problems and the other only with mental retardation problems. A physician who may serve the whole area certainly cannot partition himself and become expert in only one aspect of the problem. Rather, individuals at the local level have to be as generalized as possible so that all aspects of the mental health-retardation problem can be handled. When we move to the comprehensive centers we have to raise a different kind of question. Here, two separate facilities may at times be feasible, but they still would not be the best answer to the problem because the treatment needs of various types of patients are often very similar; the actual goals are based primarily on the level of functioning and the expectancy for improvement.

The second difficulty which exists in the development of comprehensive centers is the tendency to stay a little too close to the medical model. The essential aspect of the medical model as found in the typical clinic is that the patient comes in and the physician brings all of his medical knowledge to bear on the diagnosis. There is a thorough physical examination, there are laboratory reports, there is a history taken, all attempting to find the diagnosis of the present condition and the surrounding implications as to what might have caused it. Once this has been accomplished, if the results describe a known condition for which there is a known treatment, the treatment is instituted. If it is not a condition for which there is a known treatment, various test treatments are instituted. But either way, there are prescriptions based on the patient's going away, following the rules, and returning at a specific time. If, of course, the diagnosis proves the presence of a more severe condition, the patient may be temporarily hospitalized. There may be, for example, an immediate surgical intervention; but the treatment and what occurs is pretty much defined by the nature of the problem, and the physician does not expect to have to spend a great deal of time with the patient after the diagnosis has been made.

Now, mental health problems are almost the exact opposite, and this is what was meant in saying that the medical model would not and does not specifically apply. Quite often in these instances the diagnosis is relatively easy. For example, a child with Down's syndrome walks into a clinic and, while certain tests may be run (particularly now that we are interested in trisomy-21 and other chromosomal questions) and there may be some lab work and other things, generally speaking, the diagnosis becomes the least of our problems. What is more important is what is going to be done about this child. This involves a highly organized program of education, training, possibly amalgamated with speech therapy, possibly some occupational therapy, maybe even some play therapy, because there are emotionally disturbed children with Down's syndrome just as there are without. This means the staff members of the comprehensive center need to see their patients on a very regular basis possibly for as long as an hour at a time with a relatively high degree of frequency but with a relatively low degree of expectancy of observable changes within a short period. This is why the residential institution has remained the treatment of choice in the minds of many people. But, if we can recognize that the same kinds of treatment and training patterns just described can work effectively on a community level, then we can conceptualize comprehensive centers doing this type of job without the need of the child's sleeping and eating away from home. This is the element of the residential setting which, in terms of our interest as taxpayers, is the most expensive.

This notion of the function of comprehensive centers puts the whole problem of evaluation of the mentally retarded into a new light. Some information in terms of rehabilitation recommendations can be fed back to local facilities. Other recommendations can be carried out within the comprehensive setting. And some recommendations may be referred to more specialized settings, so that the problem of evaluation takes on many new aspects. In view of the three parts of the AAMD definition, we might at this point look at "subaverage intellectual functioning" in terms of the comprehensive center. Does this aspect of the evaluation really have any relevance for them? Does it matter to them that the child comes in with a low IQ or some other measurement deficiency? They are not going to deal with the IQ; they certainly do not plan to treat an IQ.

While it probably is important for the purpose of etiological analysis to know whether the condition "occurred during the developmental period" since this will indicate something about the extent of potential reversibility, beyond that point in the initial evaluation, this information is not important. They are going to be vitally interested, however, in the question of how the child adapts to his deficiencies, because it is the adaptive behavior which represents the reversible aspect of mental retardation. It is this aspect with which they are going to have to come to grips. For example, if the child demonstrates a learning block and is emotionally disturbed, they need to introduce him into a psychotherapy program. This will help special education in the home community to deal with the learning problem by treating (to the extent to which they are able) the emotional disturbance. Or, for another example, if the child has seizures along with a learning problem, the center will attempt to control the seizures, thus making the child a better candidate for other special procedures. The center should at the same time institute those procedures as needed. The evaluation aspects of the question in relation to subaverage intellectual functioning therefore are almost irrelevant. These are the sort of things which are known when the child enters the clinic or service, but which, beyond that point, do not represent an important aspect of rehabilitation planning. Rather, the evaluation service has to be cognizant of the total history of the child, including all of the relative factors in terms of socioeconomic origin, other areas of deprivation, and major questions of this sort. The evaluator has to become aware of the present level of functioning as defined by various measures, tests, and independent evaluation techniques. These do not necessarily have to be IQ tests, but they certainly do need to include questions of concept formation, motor skills, auditory, visual and speech skills, responses to specific cognitive stimuli, perception, etc., and these must be included in the evaluation. Also, the examiner needs to know the manner in which the child copes with his environment and how he deals with interpersonal relationships, in order to form a general picture of the child's functioning in social and community circumstances. He must have some measure of the child's adaptive behavior in terms of whether or not the child is able to demonstrate a sufficiently high level of independent functioning and whether he manifests personal and social responsibility in various situations. The examiner needs to know of any specific neurological or other medical factors interfering on an acute or chronic basis with the present potential for functioning within the child. Finally, he needs to know how these observed behaviors and symptoms compare with those of individuals of similar age, social origin, national background, etc. These are the things which have to be evaluated because, while they do not lead to a specific diagnosis or label, they do permit us to observe the child in terms of the treatment into which we intend to place him. They give some indication of how we might expect him to respond to that treatment and, more important, how we expect him to survive within the structure of that treatment.

If the child's problem is such that the comprehensive center's level of information is not great enough to deal with it; if we have tapped the known information in the field and we have come into the vast area of unknown rehabilitation procedures, then a residential institution should be considered. The residential institution should be an area of specialization where that which is not yet known can be researched, and where professional training in these areas can go forward. It should, in effect, be the behavioral laboratory for the universities. Thus, we would conceptualize in each state a pediatric center, a neurological center, a physical medicine center, a behavioral center and a geriatric center. These residential centers should have the best-trained persons available from these particular specialties working (together with their students) on the problems presented by their special groups of patients.[1] The patients would have been ad-

---

[1] Some universities have developed university-affiliated centers which, on a multi-disciplinary basis, have taken on some of the responsibility for the training of mental retardation specialists. This training is provided in a service setting and creates an additional resource for those individuals who could not be helped in the comprehensive centers.

mitted because the facilities of the local community and the comprehensive centers were not sufficient to deal with the peculiar kind of problem this different type of patient presented. Here, the weight placed upon proper evaluation becomes very clear and quite intense.

Now, in regard to the above, a point has been made of differentiating between that which is considered classification or labeling and that which we have called diagnosis. This is an extremely important point. One of the chief difficulties encountered in trying to formulate a precise definition of mental retardation is the fact that the term may be used to refer to various groups of individuals whose disabilities are dissimilar in etiology and degree of impairment. Because of this difficulty, specialists in the field have been working for years to develop a precise, usable definition which would serve the purposes of various groups.

This effort has been approached from two directions. The first underlines the need for an exact system of classification which would indicate both the etiological origins of the condition and the extent of the impairment. This bookkeeping procedure is considered necessary if we are to know the prevalence and incidence of various conditions leading to mental retardation, if we are to do careful research on cause and function, and if we are to improve our general understanding of the relationship between specific aspects of mental retardation and the total problem of social adaptation, learning and development. Thus, evaluation for the purpose of doing classification bookkeeping is extremely important and the eventual etiological and classification label is of tremendous interest to all who are working in the field. It is for this reason that continuous efforts to update the AAMD Classification Manual (1961) are going forward today in an attempt to keep up with the related research.

However, there is another function of definition, and this centers around the need for diagnosis. Diagnosis differs from classification in that it is only minimally interested in causative factors of the problem but should indicate the current functioning of the individual and suggest treatment or training which could lead to modification and/or improvement of the current behavior. To complete a diagnosis one must evaluate the problem or presenting behavior against (1) the previous history of the individual; (2) the observable level of present functioning; (3) the behaviors generally expected of children of similar age, social origin, geographical area, etc., as compared with the observed functioning; and (4) the needs of the anticipated program or area of functioning for which the child is being prepared. This latter must be seen in terms of the immediate need of the individual to remain in the community or of the long-range need to modify his behavior and improve the general level of adaptability. The latter may be either in the community, or temporarily, in an institution.

It is vital, however, to be cognizant of which aspect of the definition is being used in our evaluation procedures. Thus, it might be academically important to know the difference between a child with mental retardation and a brain lesion and a child with mental retardation without a brain lesion. But, in terms of planning a program, this differentiation may not be at all important since there is clear-cut evidence that many children who are not diagnosed with lesions nonetheless behave at a similar level of adaptive behavior as do many children with lesions. In fact, as indicated in the title of Doctor Reitan's talk, we have patients with lesions and normal intelligence who may function better than individuals without known lesions, but who have subnormal intelligence. This type of differential diagnosis raises a major question as to how to apply it to the rehabilitation, treatment and training of the retarded individual. In terms of this overview, it may be possible that we are dealing with individuals with abnormally functioning brains. Whether this abnormal brain function is due to specific cause or to a group of causes becomes in a sense a research problem. That is, can the child who has been born with a potentially normal brain but who has been subjected to intense sensory inundation of a type which has produced a chaotic response to his environment, be said at, say age six, to have a normally functioning brain? Rather, can't we say for functional purposes that this child is a brain-damaged child? The years of deprivation when he has been unable to sort out sensory cues, when he has been unable to get any specific kind of hand-to-brain guidance in terms of developing consciousness of himself as a learning being, have produced an abnormal or damaged brain. Now, having stated this, we must state that the situation is *not* irreversible. In point of fact, a great deal can and must be done regardless of the classification. This is an aspect of the problem which must be constantly underlined—the function of differential classification is not to decide whether something can be done but rather, as stated, to do the bookkeeping and to permit study of various types of individuals and their particular characteristics. We should also discover what produced their particular patterns of behavior in order to develop ways of preventing recurrence. But such classification is not to be considered diagnostic. Rather, evaluation procedures based on the way in which the child functions, the way in which he learns, the way in which he cognizes, must be developed to determine, on a priority basis, what particular learning patterns have to be reversed and which particular aspects of independent functioning have to be developed. The child can be helped to learn to cope with his environment and vise versa, so that the environment can be helped to cope with the child.

To summarize, since President Kennedy's message we have been able to come to grips with the problem in terms of the expansion of community services. It has become clear that those most in need of our help are the members of the retarded populations who are not able to find some sort of absorption into their regular communities and thus require additional support and help. It is not clear exactly what percentage these individuals represent. Parenthetically, this might even be an increasing figure because the intellectual needs of our society are increasing. We have re-evaluated the treatment and training potential of the community in terms of the development of community services as defined by existing legislation. At the same time, we have defined a different type of patient who will be seeking diagnosis and treatment as a result of these shifts in services. We have also tried to discuss the function of evaluation in terms of its classification needs on the one hand and its diagnosis needs on the other. These are the main problems which have to be tackled by a conference of this sort, at least in the eyes of this writer, who is primarily dedicated to the clinical and applied aspects of our research efforts and our treatment, training, and rehabilitation efforts.

REFERENCES

HEBER, R. (Ed.): A manual on terminology and classification in mental retardation, 2nd ed. *Am J Ment Defic (Mono. Supple.)*, *66*, 1961.

KENNEDY, J. F.: *Mental Illness and Mental Retardation*, Message to Congress, Washington, D.C., Feb. 1963.

LELAND, H.: Some thoughts on the current status of adaptive behavior, *Mental Retardation*, 2:3, pp. 171-176, 1964.

LELAND, H., AND SMITH, D. E.: *Play Therapy with Mentally Subnormal Children*. Grune and Stratton, N.Y., 1965.

NEW YORK STATE: Special census of suspected referred mental retardation, Onondaga County, N.Y. in *Mental Health Research Unit*. N.Y. State Department of Mental Hygiene, Albany, N.Y., pp. 84-127, 1955.

STEIN, ZENA AND SUSSER, M.: Mental retardation a 'cultural' syndrome, *Proceedings of the London Conference on the Scientific Study of Mental Deficiency*. London, England, Vol. 1, 1960.

DISCUSSION I

LEON LEBOVITZ, PH.D.

Dr. Leland's comments in regard to relative incidence figures from one age span to another certainly deserve further elaboration. With our accelerating drive toward automation and complete "technological" living, it is highly possible we *are* moving toward a time when significantly larger segments of the population will find themselves unemployable because of the absence of appropriate intellectual ability. Under such circumstances is it conceivable that as much as 20 per cent of the population would meet the "adaptive behavior" criterion for presence of mental retardation? And what does this portend for us in dealing with mental retardation as a societal problem?

But here we are primarily concerned with diagnostic features of mental retardation as they relate to central nervous system pathology. Dr. Leland has raised some very pertinent questions on the relationship between continuing cultural deprivation during the early years, and resultant central nervous system dysfunction.

We generally hold to the premise, first, that behavioral end results as a function of environmental (psychogenic) impingements are reversible, and second, that end results of constitutional and/or lesion-producing impingements are considered fixed and final. Yet, it may be demonstrable that one is as final as the other—or as reversible. The tremendous research (and speculative) investment in selective learning disability has resulted in the shifting of significant percentages of clinical individuals from the ranks of the mildly or marginally retarded to that of the suspected brain-damaged. It is noteworthy that the greatest percentage of individuals so categorized show primarily psychological deficit and seldom show clearly organic-structural data.

Psychological diagnostic information is "nth" order inferential data filtered through the following complexities: (1) *central nervous system structure;* (2) *unique developmental experiences;* (3) *the hardware of the tests themselves,* and (4) *the contaminations of the examiner.*

Is it possible that through refinements in psychological testing procedures and improvement in psychological evaluative skill, we may learn to differentiate between central nervous deficit reflective of true organic lesion and that which results from cultural deprivation? If this skill develops, would more accurate categorization of clientele enable us to control differential training techniques and solve the problem of reversibility?

Dr. Leland's comments relating to "boxing in" the cortex appear most appropriate. Study of the individual's concept formation ability, his sensory and perceptual skills, his coping modes, and his interpersonal relationships will do more to enable us to learn more about the reversibility or fixed nature of central impairment than myriads of classical psychometric measures of intelligence. Continued observation or treatment of selected cases in controlled clinical environments may open many unlabelled doors for us in this same direction. It slightly offends this discussant that Dr. Leland wishes to reserve this mode of evaluation to the so-called comprehensive center and away from the main stream of service, such as the special education class in the public school. If the comprehensive center accepts its responsibility and serves as part of a long-thread community-focused diagnostic process involving family and school, this concept would certainly be more palatable.

Quite obviously, the disadvantaged populations contribute more than their fair share to the incidence of mental retardation, alcoholism, tuberculosis and schizophrenia. Dr. Leland suggests there is not necessarily any specific relationships between retardation as such and membership in the deprived group. It may well be that the American Association of Mental Deficiency's statement in regard to "adaptive behavior" is most significant here. Perhaps the subcultural group is least "adaptive" and prone to produce more cases of deviant development in many directions. This "chain reaction" may be *that much more evidence* of the specific pathognomonic relationship between retardation and social class. Whether this has anything to do with "cultural" as opposed to "organic" predispositional variables is certainly a moot point. The large question is ground for investigation, however.

Dr. Edgar Doll (1941) once bemoaned the sad semantic state of affairs in this area. There was a time, he said, when all retardation was classified as idiocy, imbecility, or moronity. When you called a person an imbecile, everyone knew what you were talking about, and no one needed to define his terms. Life certainly was much more simple then, but for the retarded it held almost complete futility. Certainly, one result of our careful look at diagnostic techniques, goals of evaluation, and modes of description will be an increased sensitivity to the complexities of the mentally retarded individual's intellectual and affective functioning.

Only 18 years ago, a tremendous hue and cry throughout the psychological world was raised when Bernadine Schmitt (1946) announced she had raised the intelligence of certain retarded individuals. While Dr. Schmitt's data might have been open to question, this was not the most offensive point. Probably most disturbing was the fact she had questioned a basic tenet of our applied science. Doll's inclusive concept of mental deficiency states:

> . . . we observe that six criteria by statement or implication have been generally considered essential to an adequate definition and concept. These are:
> 1) social incompetence,
> 2) due to mental subnormality,
> 3) which has been developmentally arrested,
> 4) which obtains at maturity,
> 5) is of constitutional origin, and
> 6) is essentially incurable.

This definition placed a basically fatalistic label on any research or clinical service to the retarded by psychological scientists. Schmitt's assertions suggested something quite radical in this regard. If Dr. Leland had presented his same remarks as recently as ten years ago, he would have had difficulty finding a psychological audience. That his comments seem so "acceptable" today is an indication of how far we have come and where we are going in the immediate future.

REFERENCES

DOLL, EDGAR: The essentials of an inclusive concept of mental deficiency. *Amer J Ment Defic*, 214-219, 1941.

SCHMITT, BERNADINE: Changes in personal, social, and intellectual behavior of children, originally classified as feebleminded. *Psychol Monog*, 5:60, 1946.

II

CONCEPTUAL ISSUES IN THE EVALUATION OF BRAIN DAMAGE[1]

ALAN O. ROSS

INTRODUCTION

F OR AN APPROPRIATE FOCUS, the problems of mental retardation and brain damage will be considered from the point of view of the clinical child psychologist. The area of discourse will be children as customarily defined. There will be little said about adolescents, and nothing about those "children" who, upon closer inspection, often turn out to be forty-year-old adults confined in a State school for the mentally retarded. The emphasis on clinical child psychology further implies the focus will be primarily on the evaluation of the individual child and the planning for his future. I am what might be called a behavioral potentialist. My orientation is to study current behavior rather than speculate on its antecedents; to ask about future potential and how it might be attained, rather than agonize over present limitations and how they came to be.

One of the sources of confusion in the field with which we are here concerned seems to stem from a lack of clarity about the role the psychologist is to play. Dr. Reitan in his scholarly contribution to the 1962 volume of "Annual Review of Psychology," decried the confusion between careful research procedures and the exigencies of everyday clinical practice. We should similarly remind ourselves that the role of the neuropsychologist and the role of the clinical psychologist are quite

[1]Prepared for the Institute on Psychological Evaluation of Mental Retardation, with Particular Emphasis on Associated Brain Damage, held at The University of Tennessee College of Medicine, Memphis, Tennessee, February 23, 24, 25, 1966.

different. The neuropsychologist studies pathologic cases in order to arrive at a better understanding of brain functions. He thus, legitimately, asks what part of the brain is involved in which specific function. The clinical psychologist, on the other hand, studies pathologic cases from a diagnostic point of view, and should thus ask what a particular patient is able to do and in which functions he is impaired. Following Dr. Reitan's useful distinction of the brain as the independent and behavior as the dependent variable, one might say that the neuropsychologist is primarily interested in the former while the clinical psychologist must focus on the latter. It is when the clinical psychologist studies a patient's behavior, then begins to speculate about this patient's brain that he often gets into trouble. It will be the burden of most of my presentation to try to convince you that when a clinical child psychologist to whom a mentally retarded patient has been referred for evaluation begins to speculate about the brain of the child, his speculations may be not only irrelevant but actually against the best interest of the patient.

It should be made clear there are occasions when the clinical psychologist can make an important diagnostic contribution by drawing inferences from test behavior to brain functions. That is often the case when a disease of the brain (like a neoplasm) is suspected to be the cause of deteriorating intellectual behavior. We all know that in certain instances psychological testing is the only clue to the presence of such a lesion and that it can sometimes lead to timely neurosurgical intervention which may save a patient's life. Remember, however, that reference has been made to a *disease* process with related *behavioral deterioration* which, in the instance of the mentally retarded child, is rarely, if ever, the case. The question whether a child's mental retardation is or is not the result of perinatal brain damage is a question largely of academic interest. Similarly, in a normal child whose intellectual capacity has deteriorated following known disease or accident, discovery that the deterioration is due to brain damage becomes a redundancy. The only time when it is crucial to ask whether one is dealing with encephalopathy is in the case of the normal child whose behavior is inexplicably deteriorating.

So much for defining the boundaries of this discourse.

THE RUMPELSTILTSKIN FIXATION

The question whether a given mentally retarded child is or is not brain-damaged sometimes preoccupies psychological evaluations and staff conferences, as if everything depended on that one answer. In a well-known fairy tale, the chance for the heroine to live her life happily ever after depends on discovering the name of an ill-tempered dwarf. As a result, she goes to great lengths to learn his name and, upon doing so, earns her salvation. Many clinicians engage in similar behavior. They act as if could they but give the disease a name the patient would be saved.

This Rumpelstiltskin fixation in clinical work with mentally retarded children appears to stem from two sources. One is the disease model so prevalent in medical settings; the other is the general orientation of clinical psychologists working with adult patients. The disease model teaches us to look at disordered behavior (including disordered intelligence) as if it were the symptom of an underlying disease process. Reasoning by analogy from physical illness, one can view a low score on an intelligence test and hyperactive behavior, like a raised temperature and abdominal pain. This analogy then leads one to seek a disease in the mentally retarded child, and some clinicians seem to find comfort once they think they have established the presence of brain damage. The disease model has lately come to be questioned in the area of the so-called neuroses (Ullman and Krasner, 1965). It would seem high time that the adequacy of this analogy come under scrutiny in the field of mental retardation. If we know a child is hyperactive, distractible, and poorly socialized, or that he has trouble integrating or discriminating perceptual stimuli, we have all the information needed to plan a constructive training program for him. Saying he is brain-damaged adds nothing to the plan except pessimism, and is all the more misleading since brain damage, as Reitan (1962) has pointed out, is not a meaningful entity. Gallagher (1957) has aptly stated the educator gains far more information from the fact that a child is perceptually disturbed than from the fact that he is brain-injured.

"Brain injury," he says (and I strongly agree) "is the proper province of the neurologist but the perceptual distortions, disinhibitions and problems of association which *sometimes* occur in *some* brain-injured children are the province of the educator and psychologist" (p. 69).

The second source of this Rumpelstiltskin fixation in clinical work with mentally retarded children is the background many of us have had in work with adults. The differential diagnosis of a newly hospitalized adult patient legitimately includes the question of brain damage because of crucial differences in treatment plans, depending on the presence or absence of a newly acquired or developing brain lesion. But neither the diagnostic questions, nor the approach to psychological testing used with adults, are appropriate when one is faced with a mentally retarded child where efforts to name the disease do nothing to help him actualize his potential.

Only in a few fields encountered by the clinical psychologist is the difference between adults and children as important as in mental retardation. Many of the conceptual problems in the field seem to stem from a failure to bring a developmental point of view to bear. The unfortunate custom still used in many institutions for the mentally retarded to refer to all inmates as "children" has already been mentioned. Much of what passes as knowledge about the effects of brain damage on the behavior of children is based on studies which have completely ignored chronological age, in the mistaken belief that one only had to control mental age in order to make valid comparisons between groups. Somewhat more subtle than the current chronological age of subjects, but of equal importance, would seem to be the age at which the presumed damage was sustained, and the time lapse between that date and the date on which the evaluation takes place. A study by Belmont and Birch (1960) using a marble board task, suggests brain damage sustained by children results in a greater degree of deficit than is evidenced by adults who received brain damage as adults. To complicate matters further, there is an often-ignored interaction between age at time of damage and elapsed time since damage. As a result, test behavior will differ, depending on whether one studies a child with perinatal damage when he is four, eight or twelve years old. It will differ again, depending on whether one studies a child with traumatic injury to the brain sustained at age four when the child is eight or twelve years old; and differ yet again in studying an adult injured as a child or as an adult injured relatively recently.

A great deal of confusion also arises from the so-called "signs of organicity" derived from studies of adults with normal intelligence, whose brain damage was due either to trauma, neurologic, vascular or neoplastic disease, where there was often little or no question that their brains had been damaged. It is an entirely untenable assumption to think that signs thus developed can differentiate among children with defective intelligence where brain damage, if present, is usually congenital or perinatal, thus affecting development and not (as in adults) resulting in deterioration of previously existing functions.

Still another factor the developmental frame of reference would help us keep in mind is whether the subjects being studied live in their own homes or in institutions; and if in institutions, how long they have been there and at what age they arrived. The well-known syndrome of the hyperactive, distractible and poorly-socialized child so many have used to "diagnose" brain damage, is largely based on observations of severely retarded institutionalized individuals, some children and some adults. It is interesting that this syndrome is not at all typical in the careful study by Graham and her associates (1963) which used noninstitutionalized, brain-injured preschool children. There will be more to say about this valuable study later, but before conclusion of the introductory remarks there is one more methodological issue.

CLINICAL PSYCHOLOGY AND THE BLACK BOX

It is well for the clinical psychologist to remind himself from time to time that his only data about a patient based on observable events are those involving input and output. In the testing situation these become the test items presented, and the responses the patient gives to these items. The moment the psychologist departs from a description of these observable stimulus-response events, and draws inferences about mediating processes, he is dealing with hypothetical constructs which are no more than explanatory devices addressed to how the patient's central nervous system might operate. These hypothetical constructs, however, based as they are on correlations between input and output, permit inferences only about functions and not about structure. We can make educated guesses about how the mechanism inside the black box works, but not about how it looks. Terms like integration, differentiation, generalization, and discrimination all relate to functions; we know far too little about the anatomical basis of these functions to permit generalizations from, for example, disturbed integration to the presence of brain damage. It is much to the credit of the organizer of this institute that its title refers to mental retardation and *associated* brain damage, thus avoiding causal implications.

In a study of Rorschach signs of "organicity," Birch and Diller (1959) draw the useful distinction between the fact of anatomical destruction, which we label "brain damage," and the observation of impaired functions which *may* attend such destruction and which we should call "organicity." They stress that "brain damage" and "organicity" are terms serving to designate interdependent events, which, while overlapping, are not identical. Addressing themselves to the fact that adults with verified brain damage often do not perform on the Rorschach test in accordance with expectations based on the well-known Piotrowski signs, Birch and Diller point out this may be a consequence of the naivete of the concept of organicity. They point out:

> ". . . the concept is not a neurophysiologic concept but a behavioral one. It involves the idea that certain patternings of behavior and psychological functions exist which are the result of damage to the cerebral hemispheres. The fact of 'organicity' cannot be denied" (Birch and Diller, 1959, p. 188).

These writers point out that the notion that behavior can be correlated with *anatomical* change is inadequate, and it must be replaced by a conception of the relation of behavior to *physiological* characteristics. Behavior, they say, can be related to physiological events far better than to the facts of anatomy. Viewing organicity as one of the behavioral consequences of brain damage (a consequence primarily involving an impairment in perceptual organization) these writers conclude the presence of organicity on a perceptual test like the Rorschach is associated with brain damage, but the absence of organicity does not mean the patient necessarily has an intact brain.

> ". . . the evidence suggests that organicity in behavior is the consequence of *some* kinds of cerebral damage and not the consequence of other kinds of cerebral damage" (*ibid.*).

It is well to keep this caveat in mind later for the question of what functions might be expected to be impaired in a mentally retarded child suspected of brain damage.

The reason why it is frequently so very difficult to detect brain damage by evaluating behavior might be explained by the hypothesis advanced by Birch and Diller (1959) that damage to the cerebrum results in two different kinds of alterations in behavior. The first of these consequences they identify as "subtractive," the second is termed "additive." A subtractive dysfunction would be brought about by a lesion resulting in the loss of, or deficiency in one or more of the behavioral functions without, however, producing any active interference; thus, no such signs of "organicity" as convulsions, spasticity, perseveration, or perceptual distortions. A lesion causing additive behavioral consequences, on the other hand, would be seen as producing difficulties by adding new physiological dimensions to cerebral functioning, thus actively producing behavioral disturbances over and above whatever subtractive effects might also be operating. Individuals with lesions of this second type would manifest well-known signs of organicity, sometimes leading to such total reorganization of behavior, as was described in the classical studies of Goldstein. It is likely the many mentally retarded children who suffered brain damage in the pre- or perinatal periods have subtractive dysfunctions; i.e., they have a "mental deficit" and thus do not conform to the stereotype of the hyperactive, distractible, perceptually-disturbed child. This syndrome is more likely to be present in children who have been brain-damaged as a result of illness or trauma sometime after birth, and who have additive dysfunctions without necessarily being mentally retarded.

THE "SIGN LANGUAGE"

Attempts to develop "signs" for detection of brain damage in mentally retarded children have encountered methodological difficulties which have still not been satisfactorily resolved. Ideally, one would need a group of mentally retarded children whose brain damage has been clearly established with criteria entirely independent of the evaluations on which the "signs" are to be based; and a control group with matched intelligence whose brains are known to be intact. Furthermore, both groups must have the same kind of mental retardation. This would mean both must have been retarded since birth, for signs established on children whose retardation is post-traumatic or post-encephalitic would not necessarily be valid when applied to children with pre- or perinatal deficiences, or vice versa. The question thus arises what kind of children would be in the group of mentally retarded where brain damage is definitely known to be absent. The so-called "familial defectives" don't help because these are children where our ignorance of the reason for their retardation (rather than positive knowledge about the intactness of their brain) has been the basis of classification. Graham and Berman (1961) point out there is much doubt whether it is meaningful to speak of any mentally retarded child as being without brain injury.

This dilemma has led to the unfortunate circularity which characterizes the "Strauss syndrome," where such behavioral manifestations as hyperactivity, distractibility, aggressive-destructive outbursts and poor control are used to select the "brain-damaged" children. They are then used to validate test "signs" in the absence of clear-cut, independent criteria.

This difficulty is compounded when criterion groups for the development of "signs" are severely retarded, institutionalized children with clear-cut brain damage and such disturbances as convulsions, spasticity, or motor paralyses. When the behavioral deficits of such children are then applied in the diagnosis of a child living in his home (where brain damage is merely suspected) little more than confusion can result. It is entirely possible some of the behavior of institutionalized brain-damaged children is specific to institutionalization, either directly or as a result of the interaction between brain damage and the institutional environment. Zigler (1962) has pointed out that the brain-damaged mentally retarded and the so-called familial mentally retarded come from different socioeconomic backgrounds and family environments. As a result, institutional placement may well have differential meaning and consequences for these two groups.

Sophisticated workers in this field have come to recognize many brain-damaged children do display the organic syndrome, but that many more children who have brain damage do not fit this pattern, while others who do fit are not brain-damaged. The individual differences among brain-damaged children are so great that any generalized description of them is impossible. When a clinical psychologist, in examining an individual mentally retarded child, attempts to answer the question, "Is he or is he not brain damaged?" he must be aware he is speculating on the basis of the most rudimentary knowledge. His time and effort can more constructively be used in addressing himself to determining the child's capabilities and deficits with a view toward increasing the capabilities and overcoming the deficits. As Robinson and Robinson (1965) in their excellent new text point out:

> Indicating the mere presence or absence of brain injury on the basis of psychological evaluation is usually limited in usefulness. Insofar as neurologic diagnosis and medical treatment are concerned it is the physician who is responsible. On the other hand, the psychologist is often best equipped to appraise the assets and liabilities and the unique behavioral patterns of the child who is to be helped. If perceptual difficulties are present, as they often are, their extent and nature need clarification. Intellectual ability, capacity for expressing ideas, ability to attend to tasks, and skill in understanding and in using abstract concepts all can be explored with the use of psychological tools (p. 246).

Within this constructive frame of reference, it is possible now to turn to an examination of some of the functions often impaired in mentally retarded children suspected of brain damage. We shall look at these functions and their impairments, not from the point of view of their usefulness as signs for the detection of brain damage, but always in terms of the question— what kind of help a child with an impairment in one or more of these functions might require in order to help him function more adequately.

Manifestations of Impairment

The determination by means of psychological tests of whether a child is or is not brain-damaged is exceedingly complicated, even when the child is of normal intelligence. Functions thought to be susceptible to impairment through physical damage to the brain can also be disrupted by anxiety, motivational fluctuations, inattention, cultural deprivation and physical illness. When a child is mentally retarded, the effect of retardation on test performance is added to these factors, and deficient test performance can be caused by not comprehending the question; not hearing the question; not knowing the answer; not wanting to answer; being afraid to answer; not knowing how to word the answer; cerebral dysfunction or, for that matter, a complicated interaction of any or all of these. I shall gladly leave a discussion of the discriminative ability of psychological tests as indices of brain damage among the mentally retarded to my friend, Allan Barclay, and move to the safer ground of theoretical speculations.

Some years ago (Ross, 1959), it was my suggestion that developmental psychology might provide a theoretical framework for the diagnosis of cerebral pathology. Let us briefly review and then enlarge upon these speculations.

In the postnatal development of the child response patterns are at first global, becoming differentiated and finally integrated as maturation proceeds (Werner, 1948). Because of the epigenetic nature of development, a certain level of differentiation must have been reached before fully adaptive integration can emerge. It has already been suggested (Ross, 1955) that a lesion in any part of the brain would disrupt differentiation and integration to a greater or lesser degree and in different combinations, depending on the nature, size and location of the defect, and particularly on the developmental state of the individual at the time the injury is sustained. At least three distinctly different forms of interference with differentiation and integration can be postulated from a developmental point of view.

Integration may fail to develop, first of all, because the prerequisite level of differentiation has never been reached. This would be the case where the brain was injured before, during, or shortly after birth; this category may easily include most of the mentally retarded.

Secondly, integration may fail to reach a fully adaptive level because the brain is injured during the period of life when this function is in the process of developing. We don't know when this critical period occurs, but a possibility is that it falls somewhere between age two and seven. Many of our postencephalitic and post-traumatic cases would probably fall into this category.

Lastly, integration can be disrupted after it had been well-established for many years. This would be the case where the brain of an adult is injured. Here we often see *dis*integration of receptive-reactive behavior (Ross, 1954) in more serious cases accompanied, perhaps, by a de-differentiation, leading, at times, to the reemergence of global responses. Adults with such encephalopathies as gunshot wounds, neoplastic disease, or cerebrovascular accidents fall into this category. It should be obvious that a study of these latter cases tells little about what to expect of brain-damaged children, but it is surprising how often this simple developmental fact has been ignored.

Let us now turn to a more operational discussion of the constructs differentiation and integration. Differentiation operates when the child must hold several simultaneously-received, discrete stimuli apart in order to make an adaptive response (an adaptive response being one that his environment has defined as "correct"). A disruption of differentiation would manifest itself in an uncritical overgeneralization or an indiscriminate over-responsiveness to stimulation. These may originate internally (from other parts of the body), externally (from the environment), or from both these sources simultaneously. Inasmuch as stimuli are constantly impinging upon the organism, differentiation must be a sustained inhibitory process that, when deficient, might lead to the hyperactivity, distractibility and hyperesthesia so often described as typical of brain-injured children.

The more mature function of integration would have to be operating when an individual must combine and relate discrete stimuli so that a unified, adaptive response can occur. Our epigenetic framework would suggest that disturbed differentiation would also affect integration, since one cannot relate and combine inadequately differentiated stimuli. All of the operations generally subsumed under intelligence seem to call for integration and such deficits as figure-ground disturbance, spatial disorientation, faulty generalization, and the inability to deal with abstractions, and might thus be expected to be found in children with brain damage.

We can now briefly examine two of the most frequently mentioned cognitive disturbances thought to be associated with brain damage in pre-adolescent children: difficulties on tasks involving concept formation and in the purposive use of language.

What does that mean in terms of differentiation and integration? Mednick and Wild (1961) report a laboratory study in which they found brain-damaged children having a diminished degree of stimulus-generalization responsiveness. That is, they are unable to respond to a given stimulus in more than one way and are, concomitantly, impaired in responding to two similar stimuli in the same way. An inability to combine and relate discrete stimuli is a sign of disturbed integration; on a more molar level this would manifest itself in so-called concrete behavior and disturbed concept formations.

It would seem if a child has difficulty with stimulus generalization, he should also have difficulty in language development, where a word must come to stand for an action or object in many different situations and contexts. The often-found language disorders of brain-damaged children would thus be a derivative of faulty stimulus generalization, which, in turn, is a special case of disturbed integration. The excellent study by Gallagher

(1957), one of the few comparing brain injured and non-brain-injured mentally retarded children, reports as a major finding that the brain-injured were more deficient in the use of language. Similarly, the comparison of brain-injured and normal children in the study by Graham and her associates (Ernhart, Graham, Eichman, Marshall and Thurston, 1963) found a vocabulary scale to be one of the most discriminating of the individual tests used. Little wonder that the Illinois Test of Psycholinguistic Abilities (McCarthy and Kirk, 1961) has become known as one of the most sensitive instruments in this area.

If language is disordered in many brain-injured children, and if one recalls the crucial role of language in the socialization of the child, it is not surprising to find that next to cognitive disturbances, poor socialization is one of the most frequently reported characteristics of the brain-damaged child. In fact, Gallagher (1957) found that the most consistent differences between his brain-injured and non-brain-injured mentally retarded children were on personality ratings obtained from the teachers. These ratings included ability to postpone gratification, socialization, attention and freedom from anxiety. Gallagher attempts to explain these results by saying that the brain-injured child is unable to perceive social situations correctly, or to identify the correct social cues, or to distinguish between appropriate and inappropriate behavior. This perceptual explanation is based on his finding the brain-injured children to perform more poorly than the controls on a marble board task. It would seem that perception of figure-ground relations on a marble board are a long way from perceptions of social situations. It is true both are related to differentiation and integration. But the possibility that language mediates socialization, so that deficiency in language acquisition would precede and confound socialization problems, must also be considered.

Some support for the speculation that deficient language acquisition precedes disruption of the socialization process comes from the Graham study which, using noninstitutionalized preschool children, found language disorders in the brain-injured group, but failed to substantiate the oft-described personality syndrome. The latter may well not develop until school age, when complex social demands are brought to bear, and the child with deficient language resources and difficulty in differentiating the multitude of impinging stimuli is unable to cope with the increased stress. He now comes to manifest hyperactivity and distractibility, that is, indiscriminate responding. If this were so, then the age at which the child is tested would determine the nature of the behavior observed. The absence of impulsive, demanding, distractible and hyperactive behavior in a preschool child should not be viewed as indicating the absence of brain damage.

Before moving to the last section of this presentation, it is necessary to recapitulate my theoretical speculations insofar as they relate to the mentally retarded child. Pre- or perinatal injury to the brain disrupts differentiation which, when many and complex stimuli impinge on the child, may lead to hyperactivity and distractibility. Since adequate differentiation is a prerequisite for the development of integration, this function too will be disrupted, resulting in perceptual disturbances, faulty generalization and inability to deal with abstractions. This, in turn, should result in impaired language development; since language is crucial in the socialization of the child, the brain-damaged child would have difficulty learning to postpone gratification, and to acquire other aspects of expected social behavior. By the time a child is seven or eight years old, the interaction of all these factors would result in a complex syndrome where any one specific behavior may be overdetermined and next-to-impossible to analyze on the molar level. This may make it necessary to turn to the molecular level and the study of simple stimulus-response relationships. It is to this that the discussion will now turn.

Implications for Testing and Teaching

If there is indeed a basic function such as differentiation disrupted when a child's brain is damaged, then the closer one can come to testing and training this function, the more successful he is likely to be. As long as one deals with a second or third level derivative of the basic function, the diagnostic picture will be confounded by many interacting factors.

A strategy aimed at detecting and working with a response that is the least common denominator of the great variety of deficits found in brain-damaged children, would seem to be a fruitful answer to the dilemma raised by Robinson and Robinson (1965). They maintain the wide variety of symptoms shown by different brain-injured children requires a great store of different sorts of psychological assessment devices. They wonder how tests can be devised that sample sufficiently large segments of behavior, can be reliable, and be administered in a relatively short period of time.

In trying to help the mentally retarded child, the major emphasis must be on learning. Yet it is the tests of learning, particularly those involving the simplest stimulus response sequence, which require the greatest amount of time. The time element, however, would seem to be a totally irrelevant argument against giving what may well be the most crucial tests. I would strenuously differ with Robinson and Robinson and also with Graham and Berman (1961) who write:

> Learning normally requires repeated measures over several days and more total time than is available except where children are institutionalized . . . even half an hour is a considerable investment of time in a clinical evaluation (p. 722).

When decisions about educational plans and institutionalization are to be made, when a child's entire future is at stake, a plea that we can't afford the time it takes to give as thorough an evaluation as possible seems totally indefensible. It is difficult to imagine the parent who would refuse to bring his child to an evaluation clinic day after day and, if necessary week after week, if that is necessary, in order to decide how his child can best be helped.

One simple, but time-consuming test of a component of complex behavior was used in the previously-mentioned study by Mednick and Wild (1961) who examined stimulus generalization. Requiring integration, this function can be tested by teaching a child to make a simple motor response to a specific stimulus, then ascertaining whether a similar stimulus will also elicit that response. In the Mednick and Weil study, brain-damaged children evinced a diminished degree of stimulus-generalization responsiveness. Once such a deficit has been established for an individual child, his training program should be formulated to take this deficit into consideration. If he is to respond with the same response to two different stimuli, it would be necessary to eliminate all unessential differences in these stimuli because these would interfere with generalization. Mednick and Wild also point out an increase in drive level may augment stimulus generalization, as would a raising of the number of reinforced trials to the original stimulus. In other words, the experimental literature from the field of learning can be brought to bear on the training of brain-damaged children, once global behavior has been broken down into specific responses.

Another evaluative procedure, as time-consuming as it seems promising, was reported by Barret and Lindsley (1962). Based on the operant paradigm, this approach examines the deficits of mentally retarded children by focusing on the simple component of response differentiation, stimulus discrimination and control of overgeneralization.

The device originally designed by Ogden Lindsley consists of two lights and two plungers, one beneath each light, as well as a reinforcement delivery tray placed to the right of the plungers. Either the left light or the right light can be turned on by the automatically controlled program, and the child can pull the two plungers either separately or simultaneously. The response defined as "correct" and, therefore, the only reinforced one, is pulling the left manipulandum when the left light is on. Learning to tell the lights apart is shown when the child responds only to the left and never to the right light. This reflects the process of stimulus discrimination. Learning to tell the plungers apart, shown by always pulling the left and never the right manipulandum, reflects the establishment of response differentiation. The apparatus thus permits the separate measure of stimulus discrimination and response differentiation, both of which I have somewhat carelessly subsumed under differentiation.

When both of these functions are established, the subject will show a high rate of response to the left manipulandum when the left light is on. Absence of response differentiation is shown by a child who continues to pull both plungers, but the same child may demonstrate stimulus discrimination by pulling these plungers only when the left light is on.

> If he pulls only the left plunger irrespective of which light is on, he has formed a response differentiation but is not discriminating the lights. If he has formed the differentiation and the discrimination but continues to pull the right plunger when the right light is on he is limited by excessive reflex generalization (Barrett, 1965, p. 865).

By automatically recording all stimulus and all response events, Barrett was able to identify eight distinctly different initial response patterns and six types of terminal response patterns. These, together with differences in rate of acquisition, response rate, number, duration and distribution of pauses, and spurts of responses, permit the identification of a large variety of individual patterns.

From a diagnostic point of view, it is of interest that the response pattern on the operant apparatus was associated with the child's classroom progress. For example, the subject showing the most regular and stably maintained acquisition progressed two grade levels in one academic year, while the child who persisted in a completely random pattern for the longest period of nondifferential behavior was reported to have made no progress during three years in the same class for retarded children.

With the functional analysis demonstrated by Barrett in mind, let us once again look at hyperactivity and distractibility, thought to be so typical of the brain-injured child. Learning requires matching the correct stimulus with the correct response. If a stimulus elicits a response defined by society as "incorrect" so that reinforcement is not forthcoming, random activity should emerge, and this random response pattern may well be what we refer to as hyperactivity. Furthermore, if stimulus discrimination is defective, i.e., if a child cannot tell to which stimulus he is to make to what response, then random stimuli may come to elicit responses, resulting in a behavior pattern labelled "distractibility."

Barrett's work underscores the importance of intense long-term individual evaluation of behavior under conditions providing plenty of opportunity for each child's abilities and deficits to emerge. To be reliable, such behavior must be objectively recorded by a mechanical device, but most important, it must be appraised in terms of demonstrated modifiability under specified conditions, since modifiability, i.e., learning capacity, cannot be predicted from a brief assessment of a child's current behavior repertoire. As Barrett pointed out:

> The most heuristic description of a behavior deficit includes not only its degree of severity under known conditions but its differential reaction to various manipulations of these conditions (p. 882f).

Further:

> To select the training methods most suited to the current abilities of each child and thereby to prevent the experience of repeated failures so often encountered by both retarded students and their teachers, the component behavior involved in each task should be demonstrated rather than assumed (*Ibid.*, p. 880).

Once it has been established a child has a deficit in differentiation, various manipulations can be introduced in an attempt to help him compensate for or overcome the deficiency. Here, too, approaches derived from the operant paradigm appear to hold promise. Bijou and Baer (1963) describe a procedure for teaching the discrimination of abstract forms which can be readily expanded to include the discrimination of letters and words. Carefully designed and individualized programs taking a specific child's available response repertoire into consideration, paying attention to what reinforcers and what schedules of reinforcement are effective for him, should make it possible to teach even a severely retarded brain-injured child material which, with a more global approach, he was previously thought incapable of mastering. For example, Birnbrauer *et al.* (1965) reported the use of programmed instruction in a classroom for retarded children and give the example of an eleven-year-old, brain-damaged boy whose performance improved markedly within only five months.

Once a psychologist can bring himself to focus his attention not on the medical question of whether a child is brain-injured, but on the educational question of how to maximize the child's potential; once he shifts from looking for deficits to searching out capacities, and once he attends to the findings emerging from the psychological laboratory, bringing these to bear on his work, his contributions to the mentally retarded brain-damaged child become constructive and exciting. The notion of brain damage has long had a connotation of finality which has implied a pessimistic outlook. When the focus is shifted from damage of the brain to behavioral potential, each child presents a challenge and opportunity, not merely an exercise in classification.

1. BARRETT, BEATRICE H.: Acquisition of operant differentiation and discrimination in institutionalized retarded children. *Amer J Orthopsychiat,* 35:862-885, 1965.

2. BARRETT, BEATRICE H., AND LINDSLEY, O. R.: Deficits in acquisition of operant discrimination and differentiation shown by institutionalized retarded children. *Amer J Ment Defic,* 67:424-436, 1962.

3. BELMONT, LILLIAN, AND BIRCH, H. G.: The relation of time of life to behavioral consequence in brain damage. I. The performance of brain injured adults on the marble board test. *J Nerv Ment Dis,* 130:91-97, 1960.

4. BIJOU, S. W., AND BAER, D. M.: Some methodological contributions from a functional analysis of child development. In Lipsitt, L. P., and Spiker, C. C. (Eds.): *Advances in Child Development and Behavior.* New York, Academic, 1963, vol. 1.

5. BIRCH, H., AND DILLER, L.: Rorschach signs of organicity: a physiologic basis for perceptual disturbances. *J. Proj. Tech,* 23:184-197, 1959.

6. BIRNBRAUER, J. S.; BIJOU, S. W.; WOLF, M. M., AND KIDDER, J. D.: Programed instruction in the classroom. In Ullmann, L. P., and Krasner, L. (Eds.): *Case Studies in Behavior Modification.* New York, Holt, Rinehart and Winston, 1965.

7. ERNHART, CLAIRE B.; GRAHAM, FRANCES K.; EICHMAN, P. L.; MARSHALL, JOAN M., AND THURSTON, D.: Brain injury in the preschool child: some developmental considerations. II. Comparison of brain injured and normal children. *Psychol Monogr,* 77:11 (Whole No. 574), 1963.

8. GALLAGHER, J. J.: A comparison of brain-injured and non-brain-injured mentally retarded children on several psychological variables. *Monogr Soc Res Child Develop,* 22 (No. 2), 1957.

9. GRAHAM, FRANCES K., AND BERMAN, P. W.: Current status of behavior

tests for brain-damage in infants and preschool children. *Amer J Orthopsychiat,* 31:713-727, 1961.

10. McCarthy, J. J., and Kirk, S. A.: *Illinois Test of Psycholinguistic Abilities* (Examiners Manual). Urbana, Illinois, Institute for Research for Exceptional Children, 1961.

11. Mednick, S., A., and Wild, Cynthia: Stimulus generalization in brain damaged children. *J Consult Psychol,* 25:525-527, 1961.

12. Reitan, R. M.: Psychological deficit. In Farnsworth, P. R., McNemar, Olga, and McNemar, Q. (Eds.): *Ann Rev Psychol,* 13:415-444, 1962.

13. Robinson, H. B., and Robinson, Nancy M.: *The Mentally Retarded Child: A Psychological Approach.* New York, McGraw-Hill, 1965.

14. Ross, A. O.: Tactual perception of form by the brain-injured. *J Abnorm Soc Psychol,* 49:566-572, 1954.

15. Ross, A. O.: Integration as a basic cerebral function. *Psychol Rep,* (Monogr. Suppl. 2), 1:179-202, 1955.

16. Ross, A. O.: *The Practice of Clinical Child Psychology.* New York, Grune and Stratton, 1959.

17. Werner, H.: *Comparative Psychology of Mental Development.* Chicago, Follett, 1948.

18. Zigler, E.: Social deprivation in familial and organic retardates. *Psychol Rep,* 10:370, 1962.

DISCUSSION I

Conrad Consalvi, Ph.D.

Dr. Ross specifies his orientation as clinical in the strictest sense. One would think he is completely indifferent to anything other than the rehabilitation of his patient, until he injects something like retreating into "theoretical speculation." This is not something such clinicians do very often. However, if we keep his stated orientation in mind, everything Dr. Ross says seems tenable, with some reservations.

One of the positive aspects of Dr. Ross' presentation is the utilization of Skinnerian techniques for evaluation and training of retarded children. There is no doubt of the efficiency of the programming devices and the improvements they can effect in some cases. The analysis of molar behavior into meaningful functional elements is also of value, though the specification of useful elements is a matter for empirical study. The merit of these techniques is clear enough and requires no further elaboration.

The portion of Dr. Ross' presentation which is particularly interesting is his attitude toward the nervous system, an anti-neurological viewpoint. This position is not justifiable within the framework of behavioral science, nor is it defensible for the clinician. Dr. Ross states that once it has been determined a child is mentally deficient, speculating on neural conditions is irrelevant. This may be true, but who is to make this determination? Is it the psychologist who makes or contributes substantially to establishing this diagnosis? The psychologist typically gets such a child after the diagnosis has been made. Rather, in the case of the retardate, it is more likely to be the special education department of some school or a suitable institution.

It seems clear the psychologist usually has to determine for himself what is wrong with a child sent to him for examination. It is in the course of doing this that he is interested in whether or not there is neurological impairment. As Dr. Ross points out, if you know you have a deteriorative process, it becomes significant. Dr. Ross also acknowledges there may be an interaction between the onset of a neural disorder and the time of evaluation. If such a condition exists, one has an entirely different case than the type commonly called "familial mental deficiency" or "primary amentia." If you have a retarded child in whom you can assume the neurological state is stable, subnormal (but not likely to deteriorate) then the physical aspects are unimportant. The point is it must be considered initially in almost every case that is examined. That is, the psychologist must be sensitive to the possibility of neurological involvement, and cannot ignore the physical condition of the patient's brain.

Dr. Ross' position also has implications for behavioral science in general, though as a strict clinician, he has made no direct comments in this regard. There are indications in Dr. Ross' presentation of Skinner's (1953) notion of what psychology as a science should or should not be. This relatively recent attempt to impose limitations on psychology, particularly in regard to physiological variables, does not have any more cogency than other such attempts in the past. Forty-seven years ago, Watson (1919) attempted to stamp out the mind. For the past fifteen or twenty years, Skinner has been trying to stamp out the nervous system, trying, at least, to stamp it out of psychology. This cannot be regarded as a particularly valuable contribution to the study of behavior. Dr. Ross has a point in saying there can be a science of psychology without reductionism, but this insistence that there is no place for a physiological reductionism in psychology is without merit.

REFERENCES

SKINNER, B. F.: *Science and Human Behavior.* New York, Macmillan, 1953.
WATSON, J. B.: *Psychology from the Standpoint of a Behaviorist.* Philadelphia, Lippincott, 1919.

DISCUSSION II

PRABHA KHANNA, PH.D.

There is a need to clarify the "philosophy of science" of the issues raised by Drs. Ross and Consalvi, especially the latter's comments about Dr. Ross' being antineurological. We may like to call Dr. Ross aneourological, but we cannot call him antineurological.

Let us step back and examine the problem of types of scientific explanation as first proposed by Comte (in DeGrange, 1931) and more recently by Marx (1961). Marx arranges the various sciences along a vertical dimension, with the social sciences on top and physics at the bottom. The position of a science along this vertical dimension is determined by its unit of analysis—the more molar being above and the molecular being below. An explanation can be constructive, i.e., be concerned with the horizontal dimension of this scheme, or it can be reductive, namely, move from the molar to the molecular. Brain damage refers to special instances of the correlations between the brain and behavioral dimensions. Since neither brain functions nor behavioral functions are unidimensional, there are bound to be multicorrelations, rather than just one. Dr. Ross refers to the distinction between organicity and brain damage. In this context, organicity refers to the behavioral dimension involved in these correlations, and brain damage to the neurological. We may choose to assume the correlation or correlations exist, and merely identify one set of dimensions because of our present lack of knowledge, but at some point, the dimensions involved and the nature of the correlation have to be identified if the terms brain damage and organicity are to have any meaning.

The present discussant agrees with Dr. Ross' reference to the Rumpelstiltskin fixation. It has the properties of functional autonomy. Having started the labeling procedure, we have not really kept account of our batting averages. We do not always keep score in view of this assumed correlation just mentioned.

We would like to discuss Dr. Ross' presentation of a "theory" about discrimination and disintegration. As an arbitrary choice, he chose the instance where, as he put it, society has labeled the task as being correct or incorrect. He refers to this later in the Barrett demonstration, where there is a correct light or an incorrect light, and hypothesizes how the child's inability to make this discrimination between the two eventually leads to random behavior. One can also conceive of an instance where society does not (society in this case being the adults the child is exposed to) define the lights as being correct or incorrect. The child's task becomes harder not because there is a clear-cut positive or negative reinforcement, but because there is random reinforcement. The child's random behavior, his hyperactivity and his distractibility are then a function not of his inability to discriminate, but the adults' random behavior. This is emphasized because we have the end product of hyperactivity, and from that we are to speculate which of these conditions prevail. We ought to consider both alternatives rather than one.

Lastly, we need to emphasize Dr. Ross' point of view that we need extensive testing and should be concerned not only with status quo, but also what the child can potentially do. Lewin (1935) formulates behavior as a function of P and E ($B = f [P, E]$). Psychological testing has been too preoccupied with the P element of this equation (the personality variables) and has only sampled E in such tests as "situational tests." We need to sample not only the P but the interaction between the P and E. This applies to the mentally retarded child also, brain-damaged or non-brain-damaged. Whether or not we can settle the issue of the brain damage, we need to know what can be done with this child. We should know not only what his status quo is, but what his limits are, what kind of new situations will he react to and in which way, with the emphasis again being on the interaction between the child and the environment.

REFERENCES

DeGrange, M. Q.: The method of Auguste Comte. In Rice, S. (Ed.): *Methods in Social Science*. Chicago, University of Chicago Press, 1931, pp. 19-58.

Lewin, K.: *A Dynamic Theory of Personality*. New York, McGraw-Hill, 1935.

Marx, M. H.: *Psychological Theory: Contemporary Readings*. New York, Macmillan, 1961.

III

PSYCHOLOGICAL ASSESSMENT OF DEFICITS ASSOCIATED WITH BRAIN LESIONS IN SUBJECTS WITH NORMAL AND SUBNORMAL INTELLIGENCE[1]

RALPH M. REITAN, PH.D.

During the last thirty-five years, a number of methods have been proposed for inferring damage of the human brain from psychological test results. These methods have been used extensively not only in the attempt to reach generalizations regarding the psychological effects of brain lesions through controlled research efforts, but also in clinical assessments of individual human subjects. In fact, one or more of these methods, depending upon the particular psychological tests involved, is routinely used in nearly every psychological diagnostic clinic or service in the United States (at least in selected instances) as a basis for conclusions regarding the possibility that individual children or adults have undergone damage to the brain. An examination of the theoretical and practical strengths and weaknesses of these various methods would thus seem appropriate toward a constructive desire to improve critical standards in both research and practice.

Such an examination is presently of increased importance because of a growing inclination to apply these methods as part of a more comprehensive evaluation to determine the nature and extent of psychological changes due to brain damage, as compared with other impairing influences. Clinicians are becoming

[1]The research reported in this paper has been supported in the main by grants NB-1468 and NB-5211 from the National Institute of Neurological Diseases and Blindness and grant CD-15 from the Division of Chronic Diseases, Public Health Service.

increasingly aware that psychological deficit, particularly in children, is rarely subject to adequate explanation by postulating one-to-one relationships; i.e., a single etiological factor as the sole explanation of the deficit. While a categorical factor, such as damage to the brain through illness or injury, may initiate a process of events leading to the eventual clinical picture seen by the psychologist, it is important to realize that, in time, a host of additional influential variables are brought into play almost as an inescapable consequence of the initial impairing condition. Change begets change, and psychological impairment may well beget further psychological impairment. This would seem to be particularly true in many instances of mental retardation. Since the retarded individual may never have been able fully to appreciate normal experiences, and since environmental influences upon him themselves have almost certainly been deviant from normal influences, his eventual psychological development must certainly be a function of difficult-to-define complex and diversified factors. This rationale could serve as a preface for a discussion of the importance of early treatment of retarded or impaired persons before the adverse consequential effects of the initial causative circumstances exert their own influences. However, our present purpose is to call attention to the complexities involved in drawing inferences about the condition of the brain from psychological measurements of retarded subjects. If the available methods for drawing inferences regarding the condition of the brain are subject to theoretical and practical limitations in relatively uncomplicated instances, what are the prospects for applying such methods in the area of mental retardation? The purpose of this paper will be to review these methods and to consider, by illustration, their applicability in discerning the presence of cerebral damage in the mentally retarded.

PSYCHOLOGICAL METHODS FOR INFERRING CEREBRAL DAMAGE

Level of Performance

The level of performance of an individual or group of subjects, as compared with some type of normative standard, has frequently been used to characterize the nature and degree of deficit resulting from brain damage, or to infer the presence of brain damage. Many research studies have used the method of comparing central tendency differences (with relation to variability of groups with and without cerebral lesions) as a means of learning the types of performances which are significantly impaired by brain damage. Reports have appeared indicating very striking and highly significant intergroup mean differences on a large number and range of psychological tests. Undoubtedly, cerebral damage has a general effect of reducing many abilities. Nevertheless, the results of such studies are difficult to apply (insofar as they involve only single tests) to evaluation of individual subjects. Three factors are principally responsible for this difficulty:

A great number of variables other than brain damage have also been shown clearly and unequivocally to have an adverse effect on level of psychological test performance (e.g., genetic variables, cultural deprivation, educational disadvantages, psychotic and other emotional conditions, normal aging, and many other factors which overlap only partially, if at all, with what is usually meant by cerebral damage). Thus, a person who performs poorly may do so for a number of possible reasons other than brain damage.

The psychological deficits resulting from cerebral damage are imposed on persons of varying premorbid ability levels. Thus, a person of very superior initial ability, for example, may have sustained a pronounced loss but still be in the average range for persons without evidence of cerebral damage.

Psychological deficits resulting from cerebral damage are not necessarily constant, but may show striking intra-individual changes in time, even though the neurological diagnosis does not change. An illustration of this latter point is a rather extreme, but illuminating, example of a thirty-two-year-old woman who suffered a dissecting aneurysm of the left internal carotid artery. Angiography demonstrated complete occlusion of the artery, and a substantial portion of blood supply to the brain must have been cut off. Psychological testing at this time indicated very poor levels of performance on many tests, with a Verbal IQ of 52 and a Performance IQ of 80. Three months later, though angiograms still showed complete occlusion of the artery (but also showed some evidence of development of collateral circulation), the patient's Verbal and Performance IQ values were 105 and 110 respectively. She had not been given any formal rehabilitation program during the three-month interval. In all probability, the dramatic improvement was a reflection of the remarkable biological adaptability of the human organism as reflected in improved brain functions. The point to consider with relation to the present argument, however, is the change in level of performance over a three-month period even though the neurological diagnosis (if not the neurological condition) remained basically the same.

The first two difficulties cited above would be remedied if psychological tests existed on which deficits were consistently present and only present when cerebral damage was also present. The Halstead Impairment Index and Category Test for adult subjects are quite consistent in indicating impairment in the presence of cerebral damage (Reitan, 1955a). But there is no question that serious impairment resulting from other conditions could also result in poor scores on these measures. Thus, while false-negatives may be largely eliminated, the definite possibility of false-positives, using cerebral damage as the prediction criterion, is present. The prospect of obtaining false-positives appears essentially inescapable with any ability-measuring instrument yielding scaled, continuous score distributions.

Qualitative Deficiencies in Psychological Test Performances

Some investigators have claimed the basic deficit resulting from cerebral lesions relates to a fundamental alteration of approach or method in cognitive and intellectual processes. Essentially, this claim has stated or implied that cerebral damage causes deficits which are different in kind rather than degree from normal behavior. With respect to abstraction ability, which has been postulated as the integral aspect of intelligence (Terman, 1921), Goldstein (1940) has said: "Even in its simplest form, however, abstraction is separate in principle from concrete behavior. There is no gradual transition from one to the other" (p. 258). Goldstein (1942) has further contended that this change in "kind" of psychological function renders the quantitative results of test administration meaningless since, even if the same test is administered to normal and brain-damaged subjects, the results are not comparable. Obviously, this position is the antithesis of the approach described above, which depends upon measured differences in level of performance.

Even though the value of quantitative measurement in the

tradition of psychological evaluation is in need of no defense, Goldstein's position seemed to have such potentially devastating consequences that a series of studies was designed. These inquired specifically as to whether or not the same abilities, measured in a comparable way, were being used by persons with and without cerebral lesions (Reitan, 1956, 1957, 1958a, 1959a, 1959b).

Fifty subjects with and fifty subjects without cerebral lesions were matched in pairs for color, sex, age, and education. The groups were the same as those used in other studies (Reitan, 1955a, 1959c) showing the group without cerebral lesions to be significantly superior in level of performance on most of Halstead's tests, as well as on the Wechsler-Bellevue Scale. These quantitative differences by themselves were clearly not adequate to answer the question of differences in *kind* of mental functions in persons with and without cerebral lesions. The possibility of qualitative differences was still not tested even though the same test format was used, if the hypothesis was correct that different kinds of psychological functions existed in patients with cerebral lesions (as compared with those having normal brain functions). It seemed reasonable, however, to assume that if different kinds of abilities were used by the brain-damaged subjects, the interrelationships or correlations between various tests would differ from the interrelationships shown by the group without brain-damage. Twenty-five psychological test measures were available for each group. This number of variables provided for a total of 300 coefficients of correlation when individual tests were arranged in all possible pairs. These coefficients were converted to Fisher's "z" values, the standard error of the difference for "z" was found, and each pair of coefficients (brain damage *vs.* no brain damage) was compared for statistically significant differences. In addition, the extent of agreement by the correlation matrices for the two groups was determined by computing the correlation between them.

Variables from the Wechsler-Bellevue Scale provided ninety-one of the 300 coefficients for each group. In comparing the groups, only two of the ninety-one coefficients were "significantly" different at the .05 level of confidence. Correlation of these two arrays of coefficients was 0.79, further indicating the close agreement between the magnitude of the coefficients for groups with and without brain damage. Of the 300 coefficients, 156 represented correlations between Wechsler-Bellevue results and scores obtained on Halstead's tests. Only four of these 156 pairs of coefficients showed differences which reached the .05 confidence level. Correlation of the 156 coefficients obtained in each group yielded a coefficient of .78. In comparing the fifty-five coefficients derived from interrelationships on Halstead's battery, only one pair showed a "significant" difference, and this barely reached the .05 level of confidence. A correlation of .64 between the matrices for the groups with and without brain damage was obtained. Correlation of the matrices of the total of 300 coefficients obtained for each group yielded an "r" of .85. The results provided a strong argument that the effects of cerebral lesions are not (as claimed by Goldstein, 1940) ". . . a totally different activity of the organism . . ." but instead, seem to represent quantitative deviations from normal levels of the same kinds of abilities as measured in subjects with normal brain functions.

An additional test of this general question was studied using results on the Halstead Category Test for groups of fifty-two patients with and without brain lesions (Reitan, 1959b). Our purpose was to compare subtests 5 and 6 of the Category Test, since, even though the subject is not so informed, the subtests are based on the same organizing principle. We wished to compare the absolute number of errors on each subtest for the group, the absolute improvement shown from subtest 5 to subtest 6, and the proportional improvement. The hypothesis was that the group with brain lesions would perform more poorly on each subtest, and that possible differences in type of abstraction abilities might be reflected by differences in the absolute or proportional degree of improvement from subtest 5 to 6. We were particularly interested in testing Goldstein's (1940) contention that brain lesions caused an essential change through transforming abstraction abilities into concrete performances. Our results showed clearly significant differences between the groups with respect to the number of errors made on each subtest considered individually. However, there was no significant difference between the groups in terms of either absolute or proportional improvement from one subtest to the other. Thus, while the brain-damaged subjects consistently performed more poorly than the group without brain damage, they showed the same pattern of error scores between the two subtests.

This same type of study was performed using data from the Halstead Tactual Performance Test (Reitan, 1959a). The group with brain damage was significantly poorer in comparison of the scores obtained with the right hand, the left hand, or both hands, as well as on the total time required for the three performances. However, there were no significant differences between the groups in any instance with respect to absolute or proportional amounts of improvement. The results suggested that the essential differences were quantitative ones in terms of level of performance, rather than representing different types of performance in the two groups. Both groups showed clear improvement with practice, and the intergroup differences in this respect were not statistically significant. It should be noted these results are not relevant to interpretation of intra-individual differences obtainable in patients with lateralized cerebral lesions, but instead are referable to the general results obtained with heterogeneous groups of brain-damaged subjects. These findings suggest that qualitative changes in the nature of psychological functions do not represent a basic effect of cerebral damage, and spare us the problems of unreliability certainly attending the impressionistic description of the approach or method used in test performance as the expression of cerebral damage.

Pathognomonic "Signs" of Cerebral Damage

Specific deficiencies in performance, supposedly much more commonly associated with brain lesions than other impairing conditions, have been described in the literature. Piotrowski's ten "signs" of brain damage elicited from the Rorschach test represent one of the earlier uses of this approach (1937). Specific deficiencies of performance on the Bender-Gestalt Test (Bender, 1938) also fall in this category. Examinations for aphasia and related disorders in the use of symbols for communicational purposes must be included under this approach, since such examinations are intended to elicit specific deficits resulting from brain lesions. A great number of additional examining procedures or tests could be named in which the basic data sought are "signs" of brain damage, but the present purpose is only to identify and evaluate the method or procedure.

The "sign" approach may be differentiated from the search for qualitative deficiencies in psychological performance, even though historically both methods have depended very heavily upon subjective and impressionistic evaluation and classification of behavior. The difference is that "signs" of specific deficiencies are not basically incompatible with quantitative scaling of the deficiency. Binary classification (according to the presence or absence of a "sign") is in itself a type of scaling and, of course, would be theoretically subject to further refinement and breakdown into additional classifications eventually approaching a possible continuous distribution. Identification of the presence or absence of a "sign," therefore, does not necessarily imply a difference in "kind" of behavior as contrasted with "degree" of variation in behavior on a single dimension. The "sign" approach may be thought of as a primitive form of more refined scaling of the same deficiency. In fact, certain "signs" of brain damage have been based upon dichotomization of the distribution of a quantitative variable. For example, Piotrowski (1937) viewed the occurrence of fifteen or fewer responses on the Rorschach test as a "sign" of brain damage.

Three difficulties have accompanied the attempt diagnostically to identify and apply "signs" of brain damage. First, many of the "signs" must be identified through gross observation by the examiner. This has led, initially, to difficulties in communicating the definition of the "sign", to corresponding differences among judges of the type of deficiency required as a basis for identifying the "sign," and, consequently, to judgments expressing unreliability of the "sign" as an indicator of cerebral damage. This problem applies pointedly to Piotrowski's sign on the Rorschach test of *Impotence* (recognition by the subject of the inadequacy of a response but with inability either to improve or withdraw the response). In the writer's experience, this "sign" has been quite useful diagnostically (Aita, Reitan, and Ruth, 1947; Reitan, 1950; Reitan, 1955b) but great difficulty has been encountered in communicating its nature to others. That a single clinician has been able to distill a useful observation from his total experience is of little contribution to general knowledge. His ability to demonstrate its reliability and validity in his own hands through double-blind restrictions is of small value if he is unable to meet the scientific requirement of undistorted communication to others.

A second difficulty of the "sign" approach occurs in nonspecificity of the sign's diagnostic significance. For example, many of the supposed "signs" of cerebral damage are also found among patients with other conditions of psychological deficit. Obviously a subject might give less than fifteen responses to the Rorschach inkblots for a great number of possible reasons. In this sense the "sign" approach shares one of the basic difficulties inherent in the approach concerned with level of performance. Nevertheless, certain signs, such as specific manifestations of aphasic deficits, seem to be the result almost exclusively of cerebral damage. Even though, in selected instances, they may not cause any striking impairment in level of performance as measured, for example, by verbal subtests of the Weschler-Bellevue Scale. Under conditions of specificity of denotative significance, a "sign" of psychological deficit may prove to be of great value in supplementing the findings obtained on quantified scales of psychological measurement.

The third difficulty in using "signs" of brain damage for diagnostic inferences is, specifically, that of false-negatives. Many persons with proved cerebral disease or damage will fail to give evidence of the "signs." This is true of aphasic symptoms, specific perceptual deficiences, Rorschach test "signs," or probably any other postulated sign of brain damage. This problem may stem in part from the primitive nature of "signs" as a form of psychological scaling. If the deficit is sufficiently pronounced to be subject to reliable classification as a positive "sign," many instances will occur in which the specific impairment, even though present, is not obvious enough to the examiner to be recorded. An approach was used in this situation with good success by Wheeler and Reitan (1962) and Wheeler (1963) in a study of aphasic and perceptual "signs" of cerebral damage. They utilized the frequency of occurrence among a large number of possible "signs" as an index in the instance of individual subjects. This approach (with or without statistical weighting of individual "signs") yielded classification of subjects to their proper neurological diagnostic classifications about as well as a discriminant function analysis of twenty-four variables derived from a psychological test battery taking at least a day to administer (Wheeler, Burke and Reitan, 1963; Wheeler and Reitan, 1963). Regardless of such validity evidence, however, the initial requirement of subjective judgment of the presence or absence of the "sign" represents a definite handicap in communicability. Nevertheless, it does appear from our experience that "signs" of cerebral damage (selected with regard to their denotative specificity) may have definite value in supplementing results obtained on psychological tests yielding quantitatively scaled results.

Pre- Versus Post-damage Comparisons

In a few instances, reports have been made of direct comparisons of psychological test results obtained before brain damage had been inflicted, or early in the course of progressive disease of the brain, and results obtained after definite brain damage had been incurred. Weinstein and Teuber (1957) compared AGCT scores for sixty-two men obtained one to three years prior to brain injury with scores on a comparable form of the test obtained approximately ten years after the injury. Fifty control subjects were used who had had peripheral nerve injuries of one of the extremities. In general, better scores were obtained on the second testing for both brain-injured and control subjects. When the sixty-two brain-injured subjects were subdivided into eight groups according to estimates of the area of major involvement, " . . . only groups with lesions of the parietal or temporal lobes of the left hemisphere showed a significant decrease" (p. 1036). Interestingly, the group with left temporal lesions numbered only four, of whom two were aphasic. The authors point out: ". . . when the analyses were restricted to nonaphasics . . . the group with left temporal lesions now exhibited a gain, rather than a loss" (p. 1036). They do not indicate whether this "gain," based, in fact, on only two subjects, was statistically significant. Ten patients with lesions of the left parietotemporal area showed an even more striking loss. Omission of four aphasic subjects from this group resulted in only a slight diminution of the loss, and the group was still significantly inferior to all other groups. Although the same population had been shown by Teuber and Weinstein (1956) to be generally impaired on a hidden-figures task, they concluded: "Performance on a standardized test of 'general intelligence,' such as the AGCT, thus shows little or no change 10 years after penetrating brain wounds unless the entrance wound included the left parietotemporal region" (p. 1037).

Canter (1951) found that Army General Classification Test scores decreased about three-fourths of a standard deviation in patients with multiple sclerosis. Williams, Lubin, and Gieseking (1959) compared results obtained on the Army Classification Battery for sixty-four male subjects tested upon entry to the Army and again approximately two months after hospitalization for brain injury or disease. Approximately two-thirds of these subjects had experienced traumatic brain injuries. These investigators found that among five tests of the Army Classification Battery, verbal tests (Reading and Vocabulary, Arithmetical Reasoning, and Clerical Speed) were significantly more impaired than spatial tests (Pattern Analysis and Mechanical Aptitude). The differences between these types of tests, as pointed out by the authors, were so small they were of no practical significance. However, the average impairment was about two-thirds of a standard deviation. The authors pointed out their findings, together with other evidence, ". . . should end the myth that verbal tests such as reading and vocabulary are resistant to the effects of brain injury" (p. 304). It almost seems odd such a comment would be necessary, considering the abundant evidence that dysnomia and dyslexia result from brain lesions and that impairment in the use of language symbols generally for communicational purposes had received a great deal of attention in neurological literature long before psychological tests had even been invented!

Reitan (1960) reported comparisons of results on two patients, each tested before and after severe lateralized cerebral damage. Each patient showed pronounced impairment after brain damage, but the psychological functions principally affected were quite different, since the lesions were differently lateralized. The patient with damage of the left cerebral hemisphere was especially impaired in language and verbal functions, and the patient with right cerebral damage had his greatest difficulty with performance, manipulatory, and visuospatial tasks. Both patients also demonstrated some increased general impairment.

The advantages are obvious in comparing pre- and postbrain damage results as a method for identifying changes brought about by brain damage. In practice, however, serious difficulties arise. The first problem concerns the types of available preinjury test results. Rarely do patients with brain lesions become available who have previously been assessed with a battery of tests ideally suited for reflecting brain functions. At best, it is possible to compose groups of subjects who have had tests such as the Army General Classification Test or the Army Classification Battery. It may be noted such tests are not the instruments of choice (when choice is possible) in evaluating the psychological effects of brain lesions. While a broad variety of tests have been chosen for this purpose by various investigators, to my best knowledge these Army tests have never been included. This problem of the absence of appropriate, or for that matter any, predamage test results on individual patients, rules out this method with regard to any significant frequency of clinical application. A second problem with this method, regarding advances of knowledge in the area of brain-behavior relationships, is a corollary of the first problem. Insufficient numbers of patients have been available with known lesions susceptible to meaningful differential neurological classification. This problem may be illustrated by the instance cited above in which Weinstein and Teuber (1957) attempted to draw differential conclusions regarding the significance of aphasia with left temporal lobe lesions, when an N of only 2 was present in each group.

Differential Score Comparisons

This approach, in which comparisons are effected for the individual subject between measures presumed to be adversely affected by cerebral damage and measures presumed to be resistive to impairment, has a history dating back to the work of Babcock (1930). Many special tests or procedures have utilized this concept, inculding the Babcock Examination for Efficiency of Mental Functioning (Babcock and Levy, 1940); the Shipley Hartford-Retreat Conceptual Quotient (Shipley, 1940); The Hunt-Minnesota Test for Organic Brain Damage (Hunt, 1943); the Wechsler Deterioration Index (Wechsler, 1944); Hewson's ratios based on the Wechsler-Bellevue subtests (Hewson, 1949); the Graham-Kendall Memory for Designs Test (Graham and Kendall, 1946; Graham and Kendall, 1960).

Conflicting results of various investigations over a number of years have sometimes raised questions about sampling variability and sometimes have also called the method into question. For example, in studying results obtained with the Hunt-Minnesota Test, Hunt (1944) found striking group differentiation. However, Aita *et al.* (1947) obtained insignificant differences resulting principally from generally poor, but highly variable, scores (using Hunt's conversion tables) among the control group without brain lesions. Hunt, however, had used state-hospital patients with long-standing brain lesions in his study, whereas Aita *et al.* had used soldiers with rather recently sustained brain lesions. Similar differences in results among various investigators can be cited for other tests using the differential score approach.

Undoubtedly, much of the difficulty was contributed by sampling differences bound to arise when samples were indiscriminately composed from the wide variety of neurological conditions represented by the term "brain damage." While the effects of brain damage generally considered may be of some interest, consistencies in research findings based on relatively small samples can hardly be expected if independent variables of significant influence are allowed to vary in an entirely accidental manner. For example, a great deal of conflict among results has occurred regarding the validity of the Wechsler Deterioration Index. Reitan (1955c), however, studied the effect of left as compared with right cerebral lesions on the subtests of the Wechsler Scale and found that Block Design, (labelled as one of the tests susceptible to the effects of "brain damage") had next-to-the-highest mean of the eleven subtests in the group with lesions of the left cerebral hemisphere, but next-to-the-lowest mean for the group with right cerebral lesions. This finding suggests that Block Design scores may provide a better partial basis for applying the differential score approach to evaluation of the comparative integrity of the two cerebral hemispheres than to the more general question of whether or not cerebral damage is present.

The above discussion indicates an essential weakness of the differential score approach as it has been traditionally used. This weakness may be stated in several ways. First, it has ignored the question of general versus specific deficits associated with cerebral lesions. Secondly, it has neglected the differential influences on psychological test results of the many neurological dimensions which characterize brain lesions, such as location, type, and duration of the lesion. Finally, the method as generally used is based on the theoretical assumption that any brain lesion in any individual will manifest its principal psychological effect in the same way. An inferential method having no flexibility with respect to evaluating the many ways in which psychological deficit may be produced by cerebral lesions can hardly do justice to our concept of the brain as the organ of adaptive behavior. These criticisms do not mean that comparisons of various test scores may not be of value in postulating the types of differential deficit produced by particular brain lesions. However the differential score method used by itself, in the manner usually advocated in the literature, has serious shortcomings.

Statistical Methods of Prediction

Several attempts have been made to maximize the combined predictive potential of a battery of psychological test scores through the use of multivariate statistical methods. In attempting to make predictions about brain-damaged subjects, the discriminant function has been used. In a comparison of two groups of subjects (e.g., a non brain-damaged group and a brain-damaged group, or a group with lesions of the left cerebral hemisphere and a group with lesions of the right cerebral hemisphere) the discriminant function produces a single weighted score for each subject and an optimum, least-squares type of separation between the two sets of scores. The resulting distribution of summed, weighted scores in each comparison may be inspected for the point of minimal overlap. An individual's weighted score, falling above or below this point, categorizes him as belonging in a particular group. Wheeler *et al.* (1963) applied this method to twenty-four scores based on the eleven Wechsler-Bellevue subtests, eleven scores from Halstead's battery, and Parts A and B of the Trail-Making Test. In addition to sixty-one control subjects without evidence of cerebral dysfunction, the groups consisted of twenty-five subjects with damage of the left cerebral hemisphere, thirty-one subjects with damage of the right hemisphere, and twenty-three subjects with diffuse or bilateral cerebral involvement. Composition of the groups, of course, was based entirely on neurological findings rather than upon psychological test scores. Results indicated the following correct classification of individual subjects in accordance with the neurological criterion information: controls versus all categories of cerebral damage, 90.7 per cent; controls versus left damage, 93.0 per cent; controls versus right damage, 92.4 per cent; controls versus diffuse damage, 98.8 per cent; right versus left damage, 92.9 per cent. In spite of these impressive levels of correct prediction based on the twenty-four variable discriminant function, it is interesting to note these predictions were scarcely better than those obtained by the Halstead Impairment Index by itself. Cross-validation of the above results (Wheeler and Reitan, 1963) indicated a drop of between 10 per cent and 20 per cent from the levels of correct prediction initially found.

Discriminant function analyses have also been applied to data generated from the examination for aphasia and related sensory-perceptual deficits used in the Neuropsychology Laboratory at the Indiana University Medical Center (Wheeler, 1963). The results based on this data, expressed in terms of percentages of correct predictions, were as follows: controls versus all cerebral damage groups, 81.7 per cent; controls versus left cerebral damage, 93.4 per cent; controls versus right cerebral damage, 85.1 per cent; controls versus diffuse damage, 87.3 per cent; left versus diffuse cerebral damage, 82.2 per cent; right versus diffuse cerebral damage, 77.5 per cent; and right versus left cerebral damage, 91.3 per cent. Despite the fact this examination for aphasia and related sensory-perceptual deficits is rather brief and simple to administer, the results indicate a striking potential for differentiating these various groups of subjects.

Finally, Wheeler (1964) applied a discriminant function analysis to fewer but more complex behavior indices. He examined a selected set of variables including the Wechsler-Bellevue Verbal and Performance weighted score totals, the Halstead Impairment Index, Parts A and B of the Trail Making Test, a single prediction based on the aphasia screening test, and the age of the subject (for control purposes). The groups were composed of ninety-two subjects without evidence of brain damage, forty-seven subjects with diffuse or bilateral damage, thirty-nine subjects with damage of the left cerebral hemisphere, and forty-six subjects with damage of the right cerebral hemisphere. The results, expressed as percentages of correct prediction, were as follows: controls versus all brain-damaged groups, 83.0 per cent; left cerebral damage versus all remaining subjects, 87.5 per cent; right cerebral damage versus all remaining subjects, 85.7 per cent; and diffuse or bilateral cerebral damage versus all remaining subjects, 84.4 per cent. Each of the measures used in this study was examined individually for percentages of correct prediction, but the discriminant function was superior in all instances. Its efficiency was approached only by the Halstead Impairment Index in one comparison and by the predicted value derived from the aphasia examination in two comparisons. This seven-variable discriminant function was approximately as efficient as either of the two previous functions which included more than twenty variables each. However, the variables used in this study, based on a considerable number of subtest scores, were generally summarical in nature.

A problem in applying results, such as those described above, concerns the adequacy of the groups from which the results were obtained as generally representative samples. This problem is complicated further by the realization that much more refined groups will be needed eventually in order to obtain a detailed understanding of the effects of brain lesions. Awareness is growing that the meaningful variability within groups characterized only as "brain-damaged" is so great that generalizations about such groups are often not very informative. However, composition of groups with right, left, and diffuse cerebral damage represents only the first step toward the necessary breakdowns. We need, eventually, to know the differential psychological characteristics of a large number of neurological variables, in terms of their interactions as well as their individual significance. For example, the literature contains little information of the similarities and differences in effects on psychological measurements of neoplastic and vascular lesions, although some evidence (Reitan, 1964) has been presented that differences exist. Considering the variability existing in the pathological characteristics of neoplasms and vascular lesions alone (not to mention other categories of cerebral lesions) the problem is obviously immense. The task of composing large enough groups of representative subjects who meet increasingly refined criteria for precise neurological classification becomes a highly practical kind of consideration, since adequate material, even in a life-time of focused effort, is not likely to become available to any single investigator. Even though collaborative projects are immensely difficult to carry out satisfactorily, necessary progress in studying human brain-behavior relationships may eventually be dependent upon such an approach.

The problem is not specific to the use of multivariate methods, but does identify one of the practical difficulties in advancing knowledge of the psychological effects of brain lesions. A criticism may be levelled at the use of such procedures insofar as they attempt only to classify subjects into appropriate criterion groups. If this is the sole or principal aim, the effort is rather empty, inasmuch as it reproduces only classifications which may already be more validly achieved through use of neurological criterion information. Obviously, the eventual goal in application of multivariate methods must go beyond the aim of duplicating what is already known. The first point to be made in answer to this criticism is that recognition must be given to the fact that reproductions of inferences are based on data from a different domain—psychological, as contrasted with neurological, findings. To the extent that these two sources of data represent information of differing significance, a demonstration that the conclusions conventionally drawn from one domain may be predicted by data from the other domain (at levels which significantly exceed chance even if not perfectly) indicates a valid relationship exists between the two sources of data. Thus, studies demonstrating that subjects may be correctly classified beyond chance expectancy into neurological classifications on the basis of psychological measurements constitute a first-line type of validity evidence. The difficulty remains, however, of explaining the nature of psychological changes which characterize differentially the neurological criterion groups with which they are validly related. Only if this is achieved will the effort represent a substantive contribution to knowledge of the psychological correlates of brain lesions. Although little achievement of this type has been demonstrated at present through application of multivariate methods, several alternative approaches are possible. For example (with respect to discriminant function analysis), successive analyses may be performed based in each instance on selective use of varying combinations of predictor-variables, in order to learn something of their differential relationships to the available neurological criterion groups.

Multivariate methods may hold a good deal of promise in formal research efforts in the area of brain-behavior relationships, as well as in eventually providing a nonpermissive, objective method for evaluation of psychological test results based on individual patients.

Comparisons of Results from the Two Sides of the Body

A time-tested method for inferring disease or damage of the

central nervous system, which derives from the physical neurological examination, is concerned with unilateral deficits or disparities in function on the two sides of the body. A great advantage of this method is that it provides intra-individual comparisons, thus escaping many of the implicit problems in certain other methods of inference. For example, if a subject consistently performs poorly on the left side of the body as compared with his own performances on the right side, the findings would appear to have a biological reference point open to evaluation in the context of available knowledge of human anatomy and physiology. It is unlikely the subject would deliberately simulate such lateralized deficiencies or that he would be especially uncooperative, emotionally disturbed, or otherwise difficult to examine validly on one side of his body but not on the other. Of course, inconsistencies in performance and periodic variations in level of effort, attention and cooperation frequently occur in examination of subjects with brain lesions. Thus, application of this method requires a definition of the degree of differences in performance on the two sides of the body constituting a lateralized deficit. Even more important, both for an indication of the validity of lateralized deficits as well as for inferences regarding the neural level of the limiting lesion, is the use of a number of different tests of lateralized performances administered at different times during the examination. If, under such circumstances, the subject consistently shows impairment on the left side as compared with the right side, the problem of possible changes in attention and effort as determiners of variance is largely resolved. The problem of differentiating central and peripheral involvement depends upon the use of a battery of tests covering a range of performances rather than measuring only a single function. For example, impairment of motor strength or finger-tapping speed in an upper extremity could readily result from a recent joint sprain, muscle strain, or peripheral nerve injury. In order to avoid any inclination to attribute results from such a cause to a cerebral lesion, our approach has been to use sensory-perceptual and complex performance tests in addition to strictly motor tests. In addition, information derived from other methods of inference are of great reciprocal assistance in the total evaluation.

Some work has been directed toward establishing the validity of data derived from comparisons of lateralized performances as they relate to the effects of lateralized cerebral lesions. The first phase of a study by Reitan (1958b) showed clearly significant differences in efficiency of performance in the two upper extremities on the Halstead Tactual Performance Test and the Finger-Tapping Test. Eighteen patients with left cerebral lesions were compared with thirty patients having lesions of the right cerebral hemisphere. The groups were of approximately the same mean age and education. Only right-handed patients were used. Subjects with lesions of the left cerebral hemisphere required a mean of 8.86 minutes longer to complete the task with the right hand than with the left hand. Conversely, patients with lesions of the right cerebral hemisphere required a mean of 4.81 minutes longer with the left hand than the right hand. This difference between the groups was highly significant. Eighteen patients with left cerebral lesions and twenty-three patients with right cerebral lesions were compared in terms of the differential finger-tapping speed of the right and left hands. These groups overlapped considerably in composition with those reported just above. Again, highly significant intergroup differences were obtained. The group with right cerebral lesions tended to tap more slowly with the left hand, and the group with left cerebral lesions showed some impairment in finger-tapping speed with the right hand.

A cross-validation study was presented as part of this report (Reitan, 1958b). New groups of patients with lateralized lesions were composed, consisting of seventeen patients with left cerebral lesions and fifteen patients with right cerebral lesions. Cut-off points for both the Tactual Performance Test and the Finger-Tapping Test, regarding the degree of proficiency shown by the right as compared with the left hand, were determined from data on the initial groups described above. Use of these cut-off points, with relation to the differential level of performance of the two hands in the cross-validation groups, correctly classified sixteen of seventeen patients with left cerebral lesions and all fifteen of the patients with right cerebral lesions. Results on the Finger-Tapping Test using the same procedure were not quite as dramatic. Thirteen of the seventeen patients with left cerebral lesions and eleven of the fifteen patients with right cerebral lesions were correctly classified. While a previous study by Doehring and Reitan (1961) indicated at best a weak potential for differentiating patients with lateralized lesions on the basis of level of performance on these two tests, the latter results (using comparisons of performances with the two hands) showed very striking differences. Similar evidence was found for the lateralizing significance of sensory-perceptual functions, including tactile form recognition, tactile finger localization, and tactile, auditory, and visual unilateral perceptual deficits under conditions of bilateral simultaneous stimulation.

The major disadvantage of this approach is that some subjects with proved brain lesions will fail to show clear deficits on either side of the body, at least with the tests we have used. This finding may be a result of equivalent involvement of both cerebral hemispheres, initial deviations of skill in lateralized performances, or of many possible other reasons. However, we have observed pronounced deviations in lateralized performances in many subjects (including mental retardates) in whom there has been no neurological evidence of principal involvement of only one cerebral hemisphere. While this method has excellent potential, particularly when used in the context of other methods of inference, a good deal of investigative work is still necessary to determine its strengths and limitations.

IMPLEMENTATION OF METHODS
FOR INFERRING CEREBRAL DAMAGE

It is apparent that intrinsic theoretical limitations or deficiencies in our present state of knowledge render any one of the methods described above as inadequate. A reasonable approach, therefore, would seem to call for an exploitation of the major strengths of the various methods in a manner intended to enhance their complementary aspects and to permit their conjoint application to research and clinical problems. With respect to implementation, consideration must be given to the types of tests suitable for use of the various methods. Secondly, since the brain is viewed as the organ of adaptive behavior, an attempt must be made to obtain broad coverage in psychological measurement on the assumption that a particular cerebral lesion may impair one type of function more than another. Finally, an effort should be made in composing a psychological test battery for this purpose to select tests which, in controlled studies, reflect results validly related to the organic integrity of the brain.

The battery of tests selected for routine use in the Neuropsychology Laboratory of the Indiana University Medical Center meets each of these criteria with at least some degree of adequacy. Each of the methods for inferring psychological deficit described above may be applied, with the possible exception of evaluating changes in "kind" of psychological function. Our research investigations, as described, indicated no degree of the validity of this method using our instruments. In addition, the tests included in our battery may be applied conjointly and in a complementary manner in the evaluation and interpretation of the results for individual subjects. The battery covers a wide range of behavioral functions, including simple motor and sensory-perceptual functions; psychomotor problem-solving procedures; higher level psychological tests relating to symbolic and communicational aspects of language; the ability to deal effectively with visuo-spatial relationships in manipulatory settings; abstraction and concept-formation abilities, and general intelligence. Our approach was to attempt to sample the major areas of abilities manifested by human beings. Finally, we were more interested in a pragmatic criterion of validity in selection of tests for our battery than in fulfilling criteria of any specific or particular theoretical orientation or position which had presumed knowledge of what the psychological effects of brain lesions should be. Our efforts in this respect attempted to take cognizance of the vast neurological literature concerned with the effects of cerebral lesions in human beings, as well as the more recent literature based on the use of formal psychological tests. Thus, our battery includes examinations for aphasia, agnosia, and apraxia, as well as various sensory-perceptual deficits.

DESCRIPTION OF PSYCHOLOGICAL TEST BATTERY

The psychological test battery being used in the Neuropsychology Laboratory consists of Halstead's battery of neuropsychological tests (Halstead, 1947); Wechsler-Bellevue Scale (Form I) (Wechsler, 1944); the Trail-Making Test (Armitage, 1946; Reitan, 1955d, 1958c); an aphasia screening examination; tests of sensory-perceptual functions, and the Minnesota Multiphasic Personality Inventory (Hathaway and McKinley, 1943). Some additional tests in experimental use will not be described here. The Wechsler-Bellevue Scale and the Minnesota Multiphasic Personality Inventory, well-known instruments in general use, are familiar to most readers. While the above tests are administered to persons fifteen years of age or older, a battery, essentially similar (even though certain tests are simplified in some respects) has been developed for use with children aged nine through fourteen years. In this age group, the Wechsler Intelligence Scale for Children is used instead of the Wechsler-Bellevue Scale. Finally, an experimental battery of tests has been devised for use with children aged five through eight years. This battery again represents simplifications and modifications of some of the tests to be described. It also includes a number of other procedures devised for sampling performances from the behavioral areas represented by the battery for adults.

HALSTEAD'S NEUROPSYCHOLOGICAL TEST BATTERY
Category Test

This test utilizes a projection apparatus for presentation of 208 stimulus figures on a milk-glass screen. Below this screen, attached to the apparatus, is an answer panel containing four levers numbered from one to four. The subject is told he should depress one of these four buttons for each of the pictures appearing on the screen. Depression of any of these levers will cause either a bell or buzzer to sound, depending upon whether the lever selected is the "right" or "wrong" answer. Only one response is allowed for each item. Before the test begins, the subject is told the test is divided into seven groups of pictures, each group having a single principle running through the entire group from beginning to end. On the first item in any group, he can only guess, but as he progresses through the items of the group, the sound of bell or buzzer with each response indicates whether his guesses are correct or incorrect. In this way, the test procedure permits the subject to test one possible principle after another until a hypothesis is hit upon which is reinforced positively and consistently by the bell. The subject is never told the principle for any group regardless of the difficulty he might encounter, but the first and second groups are nearly always easily performed, even by persons with serious brain lesions. The first group requires only the matching of Arabic numerals above each of the answer levers with individual Roman numerals shown on the screen. In the second group, the subject must learn to press the lever which has a number corresponding to the number of items appearing on the screen, regardless of their content. The examiner announces the end of each group and tells the subject he is ready to proceed to the next group. The examiner points out that the principle might be the same as it has been or it might be different, but the task of the subject is to try to discern the principle. The third group of items is based on an uniqueness principle. Four figures appear in each item, and the subject must learn to depress the lever corresponding with the figure which is most different from the others. Although this group begins rather simply, it progresses to items in which one figure may differ from the others in three or more respects (such as size, shape, color, solidness of figure) while the rest of the figures differ from each other in only two respects. Additional principles are used for remaining groups of items, but the last group is represented by various items occurring at different points throughout the test. Before beginning this last group, the subject is instructed to try to remember the right answer for each picture, and give that answer as his response.

The Category Test is a relatively complex concept formation test. It requires fairly sophisticated ability in noting similarities and differences in stimulus material, postulating hypotheses which appear reasonable with respect to recurring similarities and differences in the stimulus material, testing these hypotheses with respect to positive or negative reinforcement (the bell and the buzzer) and the ability to adapt hypotheses in accordance with the reinforcement accompanying each response. While the test is not especially difficult for most normal subjects, it would seem to require competence in abstraction ability, especially since the subject is required to postulate in a structured rather than a permissive context.

Critical Flicker Frequency and Critical Flicker Frequency Deviation

In this test an electronic instrument (Strobotac) with a short flash duration is used to provide intermittent light of variable frequency. The Strobotac is housed in a specially constructed sound-proof apparatus. This test involves determination of the point at which a variably intermittent light fuses into the appearance of a steady light. The subject is required to adjust a knob until the flashing rate of the light is increased to the point of fusion and the light appears steady to him. The frequency of intermittency, in terms of cycles per second, is recorded. An additional score for the subject is obtained as an expression of deviation from this point on successive trials.

Tactual Performance Test (Time, Memory and Localization Components)

The Tactual Performance Test utilizes a modification of the Seguin-Goddard form board. The subject is blindfolded before the test begins and is not permitted to see the form board or blocks at any time. His task is to fit the blocks into their proper spaces on the board using only his preferred hand. Next, he is asked to perform the same task by using his other hand. Finally, he is asked to do the task a third time using both hands. The time recorded for each trial provides a comparison of the efficiency of performance of the two hands, but the time score for the test is based on the total time needed to complete the three trials. After the board and blocks have been put out of sight, the blindfold is removed and the subject is asked to draw a diagram of the board representing the blocks in their proper spaces. The memory component is based upon the number of blocks correctly reproduced in the drawing. Localization component is based on the number of blocks approximately correctly localized.

The Tactual Performance Test undoubtedly is a complex test in terms of its requirements. Ability in placing various shaped blocks in their proper spaces on the board depends upon tactile form discrimination, kinesthesis, coordination in movement of the upper extremities, manual dexterity, and visualization of the spatial configuration of the shapes in terms of their spatial interrelationships on the board.

Rhythm Test

The Rhythm Test is a subtest of the Seashore Test of Musical Talent. The subject is required to differentiate between thirty pairs of rhythmic beats which are sometimes the same and sometimes different. This test would appear to require alertness, sustained attention to the task, and the ability to perceive differing rhythmic sequences.

Speech Sounds Perception Test

The Speech Sounds Perception Test consists of sixty spoken nonsense words, variants of the "ee" sound presented in multiple-choice form. The test is played from a tape recorder with the intensity of sound adjusted to meet the subject's preference. The subject's task is to underline the spoken syllable, selecting it from the four alternatives printed for each item on the test form. In addition to maintaining attention through sixty items, this test requires the subject to perceive the spoken stimulus-sounds through hearing and relate these perceptions through vision to the correct configuration of letters on the test form.

Finger Oscillation Test

This test is a measure of finger-tapping speed, using first the index finger of the preferred hand, then that of the other hand. The subject is given five consecutive ten-second trials with the hand held in a constant position to assure movements of only the finger, rather than the whole hand and arm. Every effort is made to encourage the subject to tap as fast as he possibly can. This test would appear to be purely dependent upon motor speed.

Time Sense Test (Visual and Memory Components)

The Time Sense Test requires the subject to depress a key which permits a sweep-hand to rotate on the face of a clock. The subject's task is to allow the hand to rotate ten times, then stop it as close to the starting position as possible. After twenty trials, during which the subject observes the rotation of the sweep-hand on the face of the clock, the clock is turned away and the subject is asked to duplicate the visually controlled performance as closely as possible. After ten "memory" trials, a series of ten visual and memory trials are interspersed to represent a total of forty visual trials and twenty memory trials in the entire test. The score, recorded separately for each procedure, represents the amount of error made. The visual component of this test requires the subject to maintain alertness and coordinate counting from one to ten with the rotation of the clock's sweep-hand. Rather discrete visuo-motor coordination (a type of reaction time measure) is required to stop the hand's rotation in the correct position. The memory component requires estimation of the duration of time necessary for the hand to make ten revolutions, using the subject's initial perception of this interval as the reference point.

Halstead Impairment Index

The Impairment Index is a summary value based upon the ten tests in the Halstead battery (omitting the visual component of the Time Sense Test in the eleven tests described above). It is determined for an individual subject merely by counting the number of tests on which the results fall into the range characteristic of the performance of brain-damaged, rather than normal, subjects.

ADDITIONAL TESTS AS PART OF THE BATTERY

Modification of Halstead-Wepman Aphasia Screening Test (Halstead and Wepman, 1949)

This test provides a survey of possible aphasia and related deficits. The test samples the ability of the subject to name common objects; spell; identify individual numbers and letters; read; write; calculate; ennunciate; understand spoken language; identify body parts; and differentiate between right and left. The requirements of the test are organized to test various abilities to some extent, in terms of the particular sensory modalities through which the stimuli are perceived. The organization provides an opportunity for determining whether the limiting deficit is receptive or expressive in character.

Trail-Making Test

This test consists of parts "A" and "B." Part "A" consists of twenty-five circles, numbered from one to twenty-five, distributed over a white sheet of paper. The subject is required to connect the circles with a pencil-line as quickly as possible, beginning with the number one and proceeding in numerical sequence. Part "B" consists of twenty-five circles numbered from one to thirteen and lettered from A to L. The subject is required to connect the circles, alternating between numbers and letters as he proceeds in ascending sequence. The scores obtained are the number of seconds required to finish each part.

Sensory-perceptual Disturbances

Sensory Imperception

This procedure attempts to determine the accuracy with which the subject can perceive bilateral simultaneous sensory stimulation after it has already been determined that his perception of unilateral stimulation on each side is essentially intact. The procedure is used for tactile, auditory, and visual-sensory modalities in separate tests. With respect to tactile function, for example, each hand is first touched separately to determine that the subject can respond with accuracy to the hand touched. Following this, unilateral stimulation is interspersed with bilateral simultaneous stimulation. The normal response is for the subject to respond accurately with the following alternatives: right hand, left hand, or both hands. Subjects with lateralized cerebral lesions are usually able to identify unilateral stimulation correctly, but sometimes fail to respond under circumstances of bilateral simultaneous stimulation to the hand contralateral to the damaged hemisphere. Contralateral face-hand combinations are also used with single or double simultaneous stimulation as part of our standard procedure. Testing for auditory imperception makes use of an auditory stimulus achieved through rubbing the fingers together quickly and sharply in a light manner. The test is applied visually through use of a small, discrete movement of the examiner's fingers while the subject focuses on the examiner's nose. Our standard procedure calls for as minimal a stimulus as is necessary to achieve consistently correct responses to unilateral stimulation. The test for perception of bilateral simultaneous stimulation is, of course, obviated if the patient has such a serious lateralized tactile, auditory, or visual loss that he is not able to respond correctly to unilateral stimulation on the affected side. Such unilateral impairment is rarely encountered in the tactile and auditory modalities, but is not infrequently seen in instances of homonymous hemianopsia.

Tactile Finger Recognition

This procedure tests the ability of the subject to identify individual fingers on both hands after tactile stimulation. Before the examination begins, the examiner must work out a system with the patient for reporting which finger was touched. Customarily, the patient will report by number, but sometimes patients prefer to identify their fingers in other verbal terms. Although the test is given without the use of vision, it is sometimes necessary to give the patient some practice with his eyes open to be sure he is able to report reliably. Four trials are used for each finger on each hand, a total of twenty trials on each hand. The score is recorded as the number of errors.

Fingertip Number Writing Perception

This procedure requires the subject to report numbers written on the fingertips of each hand without the use of vision. Standard numbers are used and written on the fingertips in a standard sequence, with a total of four trials given for each finger.

Tactile Form Recognition

This test requires the subject to identify through touch alone pennies, nickels, and dimes tested separately in each hand. The test is also given with coins placed in each hand simultaneously. As an additional procedure for determining tactile form recognition, flat, plastic shapes (cross, square, triangle, and circle) are also used as stimulus figures, tested separately for each hand.

Results on Individual Patients

The battery of tests described above is used for adult subjects who are examined in the Neuropsychology Laboratory. Essentially the same battery, simplified in the case of some tests, is used for children aged nine through fourteen years of age. A third battery has been composed for examination of children aged five through eight years. While the same general description of the tests applies to this battery, additional modifications have been made to examine these younger children appropriately; some tests which differ in content have been added. In composing these batteries for children, an attempt was made to cover the same range of abilities and to avoid restrictions or limitations of the potential for applying the various methods of inference already described.

The battery for older children was modeled after Halstead's Neuropsychological Test Battery. We began these modifications in 1951 and, after necessary pretesting and resulting modifications, began to use the battery in a routine, standardized manner in 1953. After sufficient data had been gathered to indicate the promise and potential validity of this battery, we began to experiment with tests for younger children. A period extending from 1955 to 1958 was needed before this battery was put into final form. Thus, our experience in formal and standardized examination of older children has covered a period of more than twelve years, whereas we have studied younger children with and without brain lesions for a period of approximately eight years.

The interpretation of results for individual subjects (in terms of utilization of the various methods for inferring psychological deficits associated with brain lesions) has been presented previously for adult subjects with known cerebral lesions (Reitan, 1966a, 1966b, 1966c) and for mentally retarded subjects (Reitan, 1966b). Summaries of some of the types of adjustmental problems shown by brain-damaged children, and their relationships to neuropsychological test results, have also recently been presented (Reed, in press; Reitan, 1966d). The purpose of the examples shown below is to illustrate the range and types of impairment accompanying brain damage, the usefulness of neuropsychological evaluation even when direct neurological evidence of cerebral damage is not available, and the conjoint application of the various methods of inference to individual patients.

Mild Impairment Following Brain Trauma

This child was struck by an automobile when he was five and one-half years old. He was unconscious from this injury for sixteen hours and had a transient left hemiparesis for a short period following recovery of consciousness. At this time he was lethargic, had a continuous headache, dizziness, and had difficulty tolerating any movement whatsoever. Skull x-rays revealed a comminuted fracture of the right parietal bone, but no evidence of depression at the fracture site. The EEG showed delta waves, grade II, in both parietal areas, which were interpreted as compatible with cerebral contusion. A diagnosis was made of skull fracture and cerebral concussion and contusion. Neuropsychological examination was performed eleven months after the injury, when the child was six years of age. The results of this examination, in their original form, are quoted as follows:

> This six-year-old boy obtained a Verbal IQ of 87, Performance IQ of 90, and Full Scale IQ of 88 on the Wechsler Intelligence

Scale for Children. Inspection of scaled scores on individual subtests indicated a very striking degree of variability in level of performance, which suggests that there may have been some impairment of certain aspects of general intelligence as reflected by the low scores on certain of the subtests. For example, the subject performed very poorly on the Vocabulary subtest in comparison with either his level on other subtests or the expected average level.

The Wide Range Achievement Test yielded the following grade equivalents with respect to academic achievement: Reading, 0.7; Spelling, 0.7; Arithmetic, 1.1 grades. Since the subject has not yet started the first grade in school but is approximately ready to, the average scores would have been 1.0 grades.

Neuropsychological examination indicates mild impairment of adaptive abilities and suggests that this child has suffered some cerebral damage. Our results are fairly consistent in indicating that the left cerebral hemisphere is somewhat more involved than the right, but the overall set of test results is compatible with diffuse cerebral involvement. Results implicating the left cerebral hemisphere include the following: Although our lateral dominance measures indicate that this child is strongly right-handed, right-footed, and right-eyed, his finger tapping speed with the right hand was a little slower than the speed achieved with the left hand; strength of grip in the right hand measured only 9.0 kilograms, whereas the subject achieved a reading of 9.5 kilograms with the left hand; the subject made four errors in twenty trials in tactile finger localization on his right hand, but had scarcely any difficulty on his left hand; and the subject performed more poorly in tactile form recognition with his right hand than he did with his left hand. Although some of our findings suggested diffuse dysfunction of the right cerebral hemisphere, the consistency of the above results suggests that the left cerebral hemisphere is somewhat more involved.

Probably the effects of cerebral dysfunction on higher level abilities are not strikingly apparent in terms of everyday requirements of this child at this time. However, there is every reason to believe from our results that this child will have more difficulty in making academic progress than would be the case for normal, non-brain-injured children, especially because of the evidence of damage to the left cerebral hemisphere and prospective subtle limitations in the area of language and symbolic functions. His ability levels would seem to be sufficient to subserve relatively normal development, provided he is not permitted to get into problems with respect to academic development. If such problems develop for the child, he, in turn, may very well react with negative feelings toward the school situation and thereby limit his prospects for eventual development. We would suggest that if the parents are capable of providing understanding and patient help to this child in encouraging his interests and development of skill in academic subject matter, this should be done. If the parents are not prepared to undertake this role, some special communication to the classroom teacher should be given regarding the importance of patiently eliciting this child's abilities, rather than criticizing him for his failures. Ideally, the child should have an individual tutor to help him get started in the academic situation.

While there is a tremendous advantage in evaluating a child of this type before school has begun and before adjustmental problems have become apparent, we are not at present able to predict how well the child will do. It would be advantageous for us to examine this child again in approximately one year in order to assess his progress, using our present results as a base line for comparison.

In the instance of this child, it is apparent our inferences concerning brain damage were not based on the level of his abilities. Comparisons of performances on the two sides of the body, with consistent evidence of dysfunction on the right side, provided the major part of the relevant evidence for this conclusion.

A Problem of Behavioral Changes and their Possible Relationship to a Previous Head Injury

The parents of this fifteen-year-old boy report he has shown behavioral changes since sustaining a head injury ten months ago. He seems moody, sometimes withdrawn, and has engaged in unusual and somewhat erratic behavior. For example, several times this summer he has arisen, after the rest of the family had been asleep for several hours, and has wandered around the city. There is some question as to whether or not he may be amnesic for at least parts of these episodes. The head injury itself occurred when the patient was struck by an automobile when riding his bicycle. The car hit the back of the bicycle and the patient was thrown high in the air. He hit the windshield of the car, apparently breaking it with his head. He had a swollen area at the back of his head and was unconscious for fifteen to twenty minutes. For an unspecified additional period of time he was not very coherent. Multiple abrasions and superficial lacerations were present on his head, face, upper and lower extremities, and abdomen. Skull x-rays showed no fracture. After he had gone to bed following this accident, he slept for almost twenty-four hours. Physical examination shortly after the accident indicated the optic discs were flat and the patient had a tender area with some swelling in the right occipital location.

Because of the parents' concern, the child was brought to a neurosurgeon who in turn referred the child to the Neuropsychology Laboratory. A physical neurological examination, performed a few days before our testing, was essentially normal. EEG was also interpreted as within normal limits. Since this child was a routine referral to our Laboratory, our usual procedure of interpreting the test results without reference to the history or other procedures was followed. Our findings were as follows:

> This fifteen-year-old boy obtained a Verbal IQ in the high-average range and a Performance IQ in the lower part of the average range. Inspection of the weighted scores for the individual subtests suggests there may have been some deterioration of performance intelligence. The low scores specifically on the Picture Arrangement and Block Design subtests would be compatible with some damage of the right cerebral hemisphere.
>
> Neuropsychological examination yielded a Halstead Impairment Index of 0.6 which is consistent with mild impairment of adaptive abilities dependent upon brain functions. Several of the relationships among test results provide evidence to confirm the hypothesis from the Wechsler-Bellevue Scale regarding dysfunction of the right cerebral hemisphere. The patient was just a little slow in finger-tapping speed with his left hand as compared with his right hand, and he also had definite, though mild, evidence of impairment of finger-tip number writing perception on his left hand but had no difficulty at all on his right hand. These findings, together with evidence of mild constructional dyspraxia and the rather low scores on the Picture Arrangement and Block Design subtests of the Wechsler Scale, strongly suggest some impairment in the temporo-parietal area of the right cerebral hemisphere. The patient was relatively poor with his right hand as compared with his left hand on the Tactual Performance Test and his strength of grip in his right (preferred) hand was barely greater than in his left hand. Results of this type would not be suggestive of a focal structural lesion or of a space-occupying lesion of either cerebral hemisphere. They would be quite compatible with a hypothesis of a closed head injury

sustained sometime in the past and, in fact, are quite characteristic of expected findings in this condition.

Impairment of basic adaptive abilities is not severe. In fact, a number of performances of this boy were well within the normal range. Nevertheless, he has experienced some impairment of higher psychological functions dependent upon the organic condition of the brain, which would appear to be sufficient to manifest themselves with respect to impairment of capacity to adapt to normal problems of living. The Minnesota Multiphasic Personality Inventory provides evidence to indicate that this boy is quite distressed and upset from an emotional point of view. We would postulate that brain damage and the resulting impairment of basic adaptive abilities, though mild, are contributing factors with respect to the emotional difficulties that this child presently experiences. The evidence of emotional distress is sufficiently severe that we would recommend that this child obtain psychiatric treatment. The relative intactness of many of his basic abilities suggests that he has a good ground work from which to profit from this kind of treatment. Certainly his major problems of adjustment would presently appear to be in the affective aspects of his interpersonal and environmental adjustment.

A Problem of Academic Achievement

This fifteen-year-old boy had experienced a long-standing problem in academic achievement, but was not referred for medical and psychological evaluation until he was nearly fourteen years of age. At that time he was examined in a community child guidance clinic. Although a complete physical neurological examination was not given, the general physical examination was reported to be within normal limits. The child's grandmother reported he had experienced a "very high fever" with epileptic convulsions and dehydration shortly after birth, but he had also been subjected to extremely stressful emotional conditions in the family environment for many years. The psychological examination performed at this time included only the Wechsler Intelligence Scale for Children and the Bender Visual Motor Gestalt Test. The WISC yielded a Verbal IQ of 72, Performance IQ of 93, and Full Scale IQ of 80. The child impressed the examiner as an intensely anxious, insecure boy who was so eager to please that his own eagerness became part of his problem in performance. His deficit in the area of language and verbal functions was recognized both from the low Verbal IQ and the history of inadequate academic progress. While the possibility of brain damage as a contributory factor was mentioned, the anxiety of the child and his obvious lack of self confidence (patently apparent during the examination) were considered to be the principal factors underlying his adjustmental difficulties. A recommendation was made that the child be given remedial instruction in an atmosphere of patience, support, and reassurance so that his greatest need, the development of self confidence, could be met. If the child did not show clear improvement, a follow-up interview was arranged to take place after one year for a more detailed psychological examination to evaluate the possibility of brain damage.

The recommended program of remedial instruction in academic subjects was followed, but after one year the child was still experiencing great difficulty with reading. Therefore, he was referred to the Neuropsychology Laboratory of the Indiana University Medical Center. Our test results provided the basis for the following interpretation.

This fifteen-year-old boy obtained a Wechsler-Bellevue (Form I) Verbal IQ of 74 and a Performance IQ of 99. These results yielded a Full Scale IQ of 84. Inspection of the weighted scores for the individual subtests indicates a pronounced difference in verbal and performance intelligence, with the average weighted score for the verbal subtests being only about half the average weighted score for performance subtests. In addition, a considerable degree of scatter was present even in the verbal subtests, suggesting a very uneven development of verbal abilities.

Neuropsychological examination yielded an Impairment Index of 0.6 which is in the range characteristic of cerebral damage. Our evidence indicates that the left cerebral hemisphere is clearly more involved than the right. Indications for involvement of the left hemisphere include the fact that the patient was much poorer with his right hand than his left hand on the Tactual Performance Test. His finger-tapping speed was slower with the right hand than the left hand; his strength of grip was somewhat less with the right hand than the left hand (28.5 kilograms as compared with 30 kilograms); he had a little more difficulty in tactile finger localization on his right hand than his left hand; he had somewhat more difficulty with finger-tip number writing perception on his right hand than his left hand; and he demonstrated evidence of aphasia, Aphasic symptoms included severe spelling dyspraxia and dyslexia. The kinds of mistakes made by this patient are characteristic of aphasia, rather than only a failure to develop spelling and reading ability. The patient also showed some right-left confusion.

All of these results are perfectly consistent in implicating the left cerebral hemisphere and in addition would relate to the disparity between Verbal and Performance IQ values, since the left cerebral hemisphere is more closely related to verbal intelligence than is the right cerebral hemisphere.

In consideration of these results, it is not surprising that this patient is clearly retarded in his academic achievement. The Wide Range Achievement Test yielded the following grade equivalents: Reading, 2.1; Spelling, 1.7; and Arithmetic, 4.2. According to our records, the patient has presently completed the sixth grade, but his actual achievement level is far below this.

In many respects this child is not seriously impaired. His basic judgment appears to be relatively good, his motor functions are adequate, he shows no striking sensory-perceptual deficits, and in many performance and visuo-spatial types of problem-solving procedures, he actually does as well as the average child. The outstanding deficit relates to academic achievement and, in even a more general sense, the abilities of this child to use language symbols for communicational purposes. We would strongly urge that this child be given individual tutorial help in his schoolwork if this is at all possible. He needs a good deal of individual attention and is likely to have more problems in making academic progress than most children of borderline intelligence. The relatively good abilities shown by this child on many tasks suggest the urgency of such an approach in order for him to have a chance to become optimally self-sufficient.

Several comments should be made regarding the situation presented by this subject. First, it should not be surprising that a child with these particular ability deficits would have developed behavior patterns characterized by anxiety, insecurity, and an overwhelming desire to please. Considering that his reading and spelling abilities were approximately at the beginning of the second grade level, it is clear much of his academic experience in recent years (he was presently in the seventh grade) had been entirely beyond his grasp. In fact, one wonders sometimes at the extreme persistence shown by some of these children in their continued perseverance with attempts to perform satisfactorily in spite of the lack of success that is an integral element of so many of their efforts. Diagnosis and

treatment, framed in terms of the immediate affective characteristics of the child's behavior, are hardly appropriate to the
basic aspects of the problem. Despite the fact that no direct
neurological evidence of cerebral damage was present in this
instance, the consistency and nature of the results of neuropsychological examination argue strongly for a conclusion of
cerebral damage especially involving the left cerebral hemisphere. Thus, the basic problem of this child relates to the
social requirement of academic progress, even though he has
suffered brain damage which makes achievement of progress in
this particular area far more difficult than accomplishment in
other areas would be. Since there is no available direct treatment
of the brain damage, the solution to this child's problem must
lie in devising or developing some method or technique to help
him achieve academic skills, in spite of aptitude limited by
brain damage. Unfortunately, a precise prescription for this
purpose is not yet available. Progress in developing specific
educational methods and programs undoubtedly will be aided
by prior progress in relating neurological findings and psychological measurements. Information from these sources may provide not only for appropriate grouping of children with similar
deficits, but also hypotheses regarding the content for the types
of educational methods and programs specifically relevant.

A Problem of Discerning the Underlying Cause of Mental Retardation

This twelve-year-old girl had been the subject of extensive
medical examinations to determine the cause of her mental
retardation. The parents were both well educated and the father
was a highly competent professional person. They had noticed
the first signs of slowness in mental development when the
child was about eighteen months of age. Repeated and detailed
medical studies had been done, including general physical and
neurological examinations, x-rays for evaluation of skeletal development, ophthalmologic examinations, detailed laboratory
studies, electroencephalograms, and a pneumoencephalogram.
None of these examinations had provided any basis for explaining
the mental retardation of the patient. At five years of age the

patient had been given the Stanford-Binet (Form L) which yielded an IQ of 65 and the Performance subtests of the WISC which yielded a Performance IQ of 60. The WISC was again administered when the child was six and one-half years of age, yielding a Verbal IQ of 56, Performance IQ of 54, and Full Scale IQ of 51. The results of our examination were as follows:

At the present examination, the Wechsler Intelligence Scale for Children yielded a Verbal IQ of 47, Performance IQ of below 44, and Full Scale IQ of 39. Inspection of the scaled scores for individual subtests indicates that the performances of this child were consistently poor. Mention should be made that the lower IQ values obtained at the present time probably do not reflect any progressive deterioration of intelligence, but rather indicate that this child is not making the normal intellectual progress in accordance with the increase in her chronological age between the present time and previous examinations. The fact that she is not progressing at the rate of normal children, while not unexpected, does indicate that the apparent difference between her and children of her own age at the present time is more pronounced than it was when she was younger.

An extensive neuropsychological test battery was administered at the time of the present examination. The patient showed impairment consistently on a wide variety of tests as would be expected in consideration of the intelligence levels reported above. Thus, our results indicate that she is generally impaired in higher-level cognitive functions, and our results fail to show any areas in which her performance comes up to the normal level.

While other examinations in the past have failed to give significant indications of brain damage or dysfunction, our results rather clearly imply organic damage of the brain. These results were derived principally from comparisons of performances on the two sides of the body. This subject, although clearly right-handed, performed poorly on the left side as compared with the right side on a number of tests. For example, her strength of grip in the right upper extremity was 29.5 kilograms, but she was able to register only 23.5 kilograms in the left upper extremity. Her finger-tapping speed was also somewhat slow with the left hand as compared with the right hand. While these measures relate to motor strength and motor speed of the upper extremities, the pattern of lateralized deficiences also was present on sensory-perceptual types of tasks. For example, the patient had scarcely any difficulty in tactile finger recognition on her right hand, but made six errors in twenty trials on her left hand. In Finger-tip Symbol Writing Recognition exactly the same pattern was obtained, with the left hand showing significantly more errors than the right. Since these lateralized deficiences include both sensory-perceptual and motor types of functions, the great likelihood is that they are referrable to a lesion at the level of the right cerebral hemisphere. Some of our additional findings also implicate the left cerebral hemisphere. For example, with bilateral, simultaneous auditory stimulation, the subject had more difficulty in perceiving the stimulus to the right ear than the left ear. While these disparities rather definitely point toward impairment of brain function as the basis for the psychological deficit of this child, there is no indication in our findings of a progressive type of disease process. Conversely, our results would be compatible with a relatively static condition that is long-standing in nature.

While organic impairment of brain functions is clearly implied by our test results as a basis for the psychological impairment of this child, the psychological impairment is sufficiently generalized that it is not possible to prescribe a specific program of rehabilitation. We would recommend that the environment of the child be made as simple, specific, and concrete as possible in order to enhance understanding and effective communication. Further, every effort should be made to make her environment as stimulating and rich as possible. This child will profit from as strong an interaction with her environment as it is possible to achieve.

CONCLUSIONS

The preceding examples may be viewed only as providing hypotheses regarding future substantive contributions in the study of brain-behavior relationships in human beings. Obviously, the few patients* presented can illustrate only a few of the types of behavioral deficits and disorders associated with damage of the brain. The assumptions underlying the interpretations of the test results are themselves in need of a great deal of additional research in order to substantiate their validity and delimit the specific conditions under which they are valid. Study of similarities and differences in psychological deficit in neurological patients with known brain lesions and in mentally retarded subjects must proceed much further than it presently has. But this problem is made difficult to pursue because of the

---

*Many of the retarded subjects whose findings have provided a basis for comments made in this paper were available through the interest and cooperation of the Department of Psychological Services, Fort Wayne State Hospital and Training Center. The author wishes to acknowledge this contribution.

frequent difficulty in obtaining specific information concerning the integrity or damage of the brain in many subjects, with or without serious impairment of intelligence. Presently available results do indicate that level of ability, considered by itself, is hardly a sufficient basis for estimating the complex alterations in brain-behavior relationships which may result from uncontrolled damage to the brain resulting from disease or accident. To do justice to the problems, we must use all available methods and, if possible, devise new methods to study the complex interactions involved.

REFERENCES

1. AITA, J. A., REITAN, R. M., AND RUTH, J. M.: Rorschach's Test as a diagnostic aid in. brain injury. *Amer J Psychiat, 103*:770-779, 1947.

1a. ARMITAGE, S. G.: An analysis of certain psychological tests used for the evaluation of brain injury. *Psychol Monogr, 60*(No. 1) (Whole No. 277), 1946.

2. BABCOCK, H.: An experiment in the measurement of mental deterioration. *Arch Psychol, 18*:5-105, 1930.

3. BABCOCK, H., AND LEVY, L.: *Test and Manual of Directions; Revised Examination for Measuring the Efficiency of Mental Functioning.* Chicago, Stoelting & Co., 1940.

4. BENDER, L.: *A Visual Motor Gestalt Test and its Clinical Use.* New York, The American Orthopsychiatric Association, 1938.

5. CANTER, A. H.: Direct and indirect measures of psychological deficit in multiple sclerosis. *J Gen Psychol, 44*:3-50, 1951.

6. DOEHRING, D. G., AND REITAN, R. M.: Behavioral consequences of brain damage associated with homonymous visual field defects. *J Comp Physiol Psychol, 54*:489-492, 1961.

7. GOLDSTEIN, K.: *Human Nature.* Cambridge, Harvard, 1940.

8. GOLDSTEIN, K.: The two ways of adjustment of the organism to cerebral defects. *Mount Sinai Hospital, 9*:504-513, 1942.

8a. GRAHAM, F. K., AND KENDALL, B.: Performance of brain-damaged cases on a memory for designs test. *J Abnorm Soc Psychol, 41*:303-314, 1946.

8b. GRAHAM, F. K., AND KENDALL, B. S.: Memory-for Designs Test: Revised General Manual. *Percept Motor Skills, 11*:147-188, 1960.

8c. HALSTEAD, W. C.: *Brain and Intelligence.* Chicago, U of Chicago, 1947.

8d. HALSTEAD, W. C., AND WEPMAN, J. M.: The Halstead-Wepman aphasia screening test. *J Speech Hearing Dis, 14*:9-15, 1949.

8e. HATHAWAY, S. R., AND MCKINLEY, J. C.: *Manual for the Minnesota Multiphasic Personality Inventory.* Minneapolis, U of Minn., 1943.

8f. HEWSON, L. R.: The Wechsler-Bellevue Scale and the substitution test as aids in neuropsychiatric diagnosis. *J Nerv Ment Dis, 109*:158-266, 1949.

8g. HUNT, H. F.: A practical clinical test for organic brain damage. *J App Psychol, 27*:375-386, 1943.

8h. HUNT, H. F.: A note on the clinical use of the Hunt-Minnesota Test for organic brain damage. *J App Psychol, 28*:175-178, 1944.

9. PIOTROWSKI, Z.: The Rorschach ink-blot method in organic disturbances of the central nervous system. *J Nerv Ment Dis, 86*:525-537, 1937.

10. REED, H. B. C.: The use of psychological tests in diagnosing brain damage in school age children. *Proceedings of the First Professional Workshop in the Diagnosis of Brain Damage in School Age Children,* Peabody College, Nashville, Tennessee, August, 1965. In press.

11. REITAN, R. M.: Relationships of certain Rorschach Test indicators to the abstraction and power factors of biological intelligence. Unpublished doctoral dissertation, University of Chicago, 1950.

12. REITAN, R. M.: An investigation of the validity of Halstead's measures of biological intelligence. *Arch Neurol Psychiat, 73*:28-35, 1955a.

13. REITAN, R. M.: Validity of Rorschach Test as measure of psychological effects of brain damage. *Arch Neurol Psychiat, 73*:445-451, 1955b.

14. REITAN, R. M.: Certain differential effects of left and right cerebral lesions in human adults. *J Comp Physiol Psychol, 48*:474-477, 1955c.

14a. REITAN, R. M.: The relation of the Trail-Making Test to organic brain-damage. *J Consult Psychol, 19*:393-394, 1955d.

15. REITAN, R. M.: Investigation of relationships between "psychometric" and "biological" intelligence. *J Nerv Ment Dis, 123*:536-541, 1956.

16. REITAN, R. M.: The comparative significance of qualitative and quantitative psychological changes with brain damage. *Proc 15th Int Congr Psychol,* 214-215, 1957.

17. REITAN, R. M.: Qualitative versus quantitative mental changes following brain damage. *J Psychol, 46*:339-346, 1958a.

18. REITAN, R. M.: Symposium: Contribution of physiological psychology to clinical inferences. Presented at Midwest Psychology Association Meeting, Detroit, Michigan, May, 1958b.

18a. REITAN, R. M.: The validity of the Trail-Making Test as an indicator of organic brain-damage. *Percept Motor Skills, 8*:271-276, 1958c.

19. REITAN, R. M.: Effects of brain damage on a psychomotor problem-solving task. *Percep Motor Skills, 9*:211-215, 1959a.

20. REITAN, R. M.: Impairment of abstraction ability in brain damage: Quantitative versus qualitative changes. *J Psychol, 48*:97-102, 1959b.

21. REITAN, R. M.: The comparative effects of brain damage on the Halstead Impairment Index and the Wechsler-Bellevue Scale. *J Clin Psychol, 15*:281-285, 1959c.

22. REITAN, R. M.: The significance of dysphasia for intelligence and adaptive abilities. *J Psychol, 50*:355-376, 1960.

23. REITAN, R. M.: Psychological deficits resulting from cerebral lesions in man. In Warren, J. M., and Akert, K. A. (Eds.): *The Frontal Granular Cortex and Behavior.* New York, McGraw-Hill, 1964.

24. REITAN, R. M.: Problems and prospects in studying the psychological correlates of brain lesions. *Cortex, 2*:127-154, 1966.

25. REITAN, R. M.: A research program on the psychological effects of brain lesions in human beings. In Ellis, N. R. (Ed.): *International Review of Research in Mental Retardation.* New York, Academic Press. In press.

26. REITAN, R. .M: Diagnostic inferences of brain lesions based on psychological test results. *Canad Psychol.* In press.

27. REITAN, R. M.: The needs of teachers for specialized information in the area of neuropsychology. *Proceedings of the Seminar on Standards for the Preparation of Teachers of Brain Injured Children,* Syracuse University, Washington, D.C., October, 1965. In press.

28. SHIPLEY, W. C.: A self-administering scale for measuring intellectual impairment and deterioration. *J Psychol, 9*:371-377, 1940.

29. TERMAN, L. M.: Intelligence and its measurements: a symposium. *J Educ Psychol, 12*:123-147, 1921.

30. TEUBER, H. L., AND WEINSTEIN, S.: Ability to discover hidden figures after cerebral lesions. *Arch Neurol Psychiat, 76*:369-379, 1956.

30a. WECHSLER, D.: *The Measurement of Adult Intelligence,* 3rd ed. Baltimore, Williams & Wilkins, 1944.

31. WEINSTEIN, S., AND TEUBER, H. L.: Effects of penetrating brain injury on intelligence test scores. *Science, 125*:1036-1037, 1957.

32. WHEELER, L.: Predictions of brain-damage from an aphasia screening test; an application of discriminant functions and a comparison with a non-linear method of analysis. *Percept Motor Skills,* Monograph Supplement 1-V17, *17*:63-80, 1963.

33. WHEELER, L.: Complex behavioral indices weighted by linear discriminant functions for the prediction of cerebral damage. *Percept Motor Skills,* Monograph Supplement 4-V19, *19*:907-923, 1964.

34. WHEELER, L., BURKE, C. J., AND REITAN, R. M.: An application of discriminant functions to the problem of predicting brain damage using behavioral variables. *Percept Motor Skills,* Monograph Supplement, *16*:417-440, 1963.

35. WHEELER, L., AND REITAN, R. M.: The presence and laterality of brain damage predicted from responses to a short aphasia screening test. *Percept Motor Skills*, 15:783-799, 1962.

36. WHEELER, L., AND REITAN, R. M.: Discriminant functions applied to the problem of predicting cerebral damage from behavioral tests; a cross validation study. *Percept Motor Skills*, 16:681-701, 1963.

37. WILLIAMS, H. L., LUBIN, A., AND GIESEKING, C. F.: Direct measurement of cognitive deficit in brain-injured patients. *J Consult Psychol*, 23:300-305, 1959.

DISCUSSION I

R. A. UTTERBACK, M.D.

There were three points derived from Dr. Reitan's paper. The first point is the impossibility of doing a proper evaluation just by mechanical testing and adding up of scores. The discriminative skill of an experienced and sophisticated observer is necessary, both in the choice of tests to be administered to the individual and in the interpretation of these tests. This is evidenced in some of the cases cited by Dr. Reitan. Secondly, it was implied that much of the work in psychology (especially as related to neuropsychology) has been based on information derived from the neurological examination in the broad sense, including the examination of the brain at post mortem, electroencephalograms and pneumoencephalograms. This has often been used as the standard of reference for the psychologist to determine how well his tests have identified disease processes. It seems the need is for the psychologist to pass this stage, and to devise and perfect tests allowing him to recognize changes too subtle for us to pick up with the tests just mentioned. This is being done by some of our most skilled colleagues, but there is much yet to accomplish. The third point is along much the same line. Dr. Reitan has strongly requested, if not actually demanded, higher goals in psychological testing of the brain-damaged; this means not only the child, but the adult who has had structural damage to his brain. There is surely much more to be learned from this technique and much which will be not only of practical, clinical value, but also of research potential.

A neurologist needs assistance from psychologists in several areas, but particularly in "screening," in helping to divert to the neurologist (or the psychiatrist when need be) the individual who needs assistance. Psychologists are able, at times, to separate the person who has structural disease from the patient with functional disease more reliably than the general practitioner, the usual source of referral. Certainly the psychologist can do it better than the school teacher or the industrial physician and many other sources. Possibly, in the future, the psychologist will be more and more able to recognize those subtle implications of brain damage so related to "higher" integrative functions which our gross tests fail to recognize. Another function of the psychologist is to help predict the potential for the patient.

Another case exemplifies the point. A child was sent to a neurologist because he was not learning well in school. It was a psychologist within the school system who suggested this youngster had a structural reason for not doing well scholastically. His mother was much perturbed because of her fear it was something she was doing (or not doing) which was responsible for this youngster's failure. She had several other children, all doing well, but this one was not. The psychometric tests had indicated there might be a structural reason for it. On the neurological examination no abnormality could be found; there was no gross defect of function. The electroencephalogram, however, showed quite clear evidence of abnormality in the posterior portion of the left cerebral hemisphere—the area primarily concerned with recognition of words and the formation of speech. In taking a careful history from the mother, information was obtained that this youngster, in contrast with her other children, had been the product of a very long and arduous labor, had required a great deal of forceps manipulation and had gotten off to a bad start at birth. Actually, no specific damage to the brain was known; he had developed at about the same rate as her other children in learning to walk and to talk. It seemed all this information could be combined to understand his problem: the history, the EEG findings, that the child was not doing well in reading and writing and expressing himself, along with the psychometric examination. We can say with fair confidence this youngster has a lesion in the left cerebral hemisphere, which produces a real, physical handicap. It is always going to be difficult for him to learn these skills. Of course, the neurologist cannot "fix" this, and the psychologist cannot "fix" it, but the boy will now be placed in a special class in school where special attention will be given to his particular problem. That may or may not help a great deal. Incidentally, his mother was tremendously relieved to know she was not guilty of mistreating this child. Possibly his teachers may also feel some relief in knowing his troubles were not due to failure on their part.

There are a few things which seem important in interpreting psychometric tests, considerations that sometimes are overlooked, particularly for the kind of patients a neurologist sees. The first is that psychometric tests cannot be done properly immediately after the patient has had a convulsive seizure. Postpone the testing if the patient has had a seizure in the last twenty-four hours. Second, it is important to make certain the patient is not having "little seizures"—not referring to *petit mal,* because *petit mal* attacks do not interfere very much with performance. Many patients, though, have momentary paroxysms of abnormal cortical discharges which confuse them for a few moments without actually having a clinically recognizable seizure. This sometimes accounts for confusing variations in test results. Third, it is important the patient being tested not be intoxicated, particularly by his medication. Unfortunately, neurologists and psychiatrists sometimes are themselves responsible for this intoxication, especially with anticonvulsant medication. Of course, patients may also be intrinsically poisoned by uremia, by hepatic failure, etc. Finally, it is important to avoid testing during a period of cerebral edema, if you want to have reliable results. This is most commonly a problem after trauma or a stroke, but many injuries to the nervous system produce edema which may last for many days and interfere with the testing results.

Dr. Reitan has spelled out some very important rules and advice for further development in psychometric testing.

DISCUSSION II
GERALD R. PASCAL, PH.D.

The measurement and prediction of human capacity is an

area of endeavor of ever-increasing importance. Factual, quantitative data in this area are not only important for the treatment of mental retardation, but also important for prevention. It is worth noting that in this area of many empirical studies, there is not one unifying theory relating brain anatomy and physiology to behavior. The systematic collection of psychological data may one day help to form such a theory.

It is evident from Dr. Reitan's paper that we have come a long way from simple measures of reaction time and the simple IQ tests of Binet and Simon. Unfortunately, however, in estimating intellectual capacity, we are still saddled with a number of ways which are dependent upon variables which fluctuate with such things as culture, mood and other vagaries of human nature. It is interesting that most of the tests used by Dr. Reitan in his battery are relatively culture-free; nor are his evaluations particularly dependent upon verbal ability except when verbal ability itself is an object of measurement. We still have some distance to go in this direction, however. Consider, for instance, the examination of a cerebral palsy patient who is spastic, and who cannot speak or hear. Ordinary measures of intellectual capacity are difficult to apply to such a person. Yet, he can be examined if we use methods derived from the experimental laboratory. The child in question could be tested on delayed reaction problems, and single and double alternation problems. If the child can move his eyes, he can be examined (Pascal and Jenkins, 1959). There are a number of such biologically sound measures which should be developed. A problem for research is to develop measurements of capacity that could be applied equally to an Australian bushman or a citizen of New York City.

Another line of development emerging from Dr. Reitan's paper has to do with our escape from the early notions of human faculties as a basis for measurement. Dr. Reitan's approach attacks directly the input and output mechanisms of human functioning. His tests systematically sample all the sensory modalities. He does, however, leave out taste, smell and proprioception. It is not known what the data are on these sensory modalities as they may relate to overall intellectual capacity. It is doubtful whether the senses of taste and smell have any relation to intellectual capacity in the meaning of its adaptive aspects in our culture except, perhaps, for tea-tasting and similar experiences. Kinesthesis, however, may have a relation. The Montessori method suggests that the addition of kinesthesis to the other sensory modalities adds something to learning ability. Perhaps we need to study the kinesthetic sense. It could be that a mental defective child, as measured by our current tests, might turn out to be a kinesthetic genius! It is hard to think what that might do for him, but it may be that the kinesthetic sense could be an avenue for learning.

A great need, as implied by Dr. Reitan, is for developmental data, using measures which tap the various sensory modalities. We need expectancy levels for various age groups on each one of the sensory modalities. We probably also need more detailed studies of individual modalities, such as the visual sense. We not only need expectancy levels for visual discrimination, but also for visual memory and visual comprehension. If we had such data for children, a good deal of difficulty in school work could be avoided for some children. It has been shown, and found to be true in clinical practice, that children with reading disabilities very often have a deficiency in visual comprehension. (At one time, we might have called it a deficiency in visual imagery.) If we could detect these children at preschool age, we could save them many problems. Children with difficulty in visual comprehension can be taught to read by conditioning techniques, using their hearing as a sensory input for what they see.

We need to know, in examining intellectual capacity, the effects of emotional factors on test performance. We need to know how to measure and weigh emotional factors affecting test performance. A child having difficulty in visual comprehension, and who thus becomes a reading disability case, gets something added to his reading disability by the time he gets to the third grade. He has had two years of not being able to keep up with his peers. He begins to "quit." At the time of examination, there is not only the difficulty in visual comprehension, but also the effects of these added emotional factors. All too often, clinical psychologists suffer from the experimenter effect (Kintz *et al.*, 1965). They tend to see in the dynamics underlying the child's emotional problem that which they want to see. Therefore, reading disabilities very often are blamed on the emotional problems existing within the family, rather than on the difficulty with visual comprehension that the child actually has. Those who have spent some time in institutions for the mentally retarded are familiar with the frequent discovery of the autistic child who was called mentally defective. In the examination of the mentally retarded, therefore, it is necessary to know and be able to measure that which can be attributed to emotional factors and which can be reversed. In making such measures, we need to be very conscious of the fact that experimental effects, such as early stimulus deprivation, may also lead to irreversible psychological deficit.

It is the proper function of the psychologist to measure input and output. A given organism can be described in terms of stimuli and responses to these stimuli. If psychologists go about these measures trying as much as possible to be biologically sound, they have done their part. Too much concern with brain anatomy and brain physiology might, in a sense, interfere with the psychological measurement process. Psychology can make its greatest contribution by concentrating on these measures without particular concern for the areas of neurology and physiology. If the psychologists find a defect in visual functioning without physical indications of it, then it is up to the neurologist to incorporate this datum into his sphere of research.

There is no implication intended that psychological tests should not be used as an aid in the detection of, and as measurement of the effects of, trauma to the brain, neoplasms, etc.; rather, that there is a place for *psychological* theorizing, particularly in relatively intact mental defectives. Specific behavioral measurements should show individual differences in mental defectives. The categorizations we now have, both medical and psychological, are not heuristic. Extension of the work Dr. Reitan is doing will lead to psychological theorizing which will eventuate in a better understanding of mental deficiency and a more systematic approach to its prevention and treatment.

Dr. Reitan's paper demonstrates the expertise necessary in

psychological evaluation. The IQ tester can sometimes do considerable harm. Proper psychological diagnosis takes considerably more than that obtained by taking a course in IQ testing.

REFERENCES

KINTZ, B. L., DELPRATO, D. J., METTEE, D. R., PERSONS, C. E., AND SCHAPPE, R. H.: The experimenter effect. *Psychol Bull, 63*(No. 4):223-232, 1965.

PASCAL, G. R., AND JENKINS, W. O.: The Hunter-Pascal Concept Formation Test: An experimental approach to the measurement of cortical capacity. *J Clin Psychol, 15*:159-163, 1959.

IV

THE DISCRIMINATIVE VALIDITY
OF PSYCHOLOGICAL TESTS AS INDICES
OF BRAIN DAMAGE IN THE RETARDED CHILD

A. BARCLAY

INTRODUCTION

THE PURPOSE of this paper is to explore certain aspects of the validity of current tests of organicity as applied to retarded children, and to explore certain of the implications posed by the resultant findings. At the outset let me point out I do not claim competence as a research scientist in the vagaries of brain function; rather, I am interested in the problem from the point of view of the clinical consumer. It is in this capacity I am frequently confronted with the vexing question of whether a given child is or is not brain-damaged and, if so, to what degree and in what manner. I have been frequently impressed, as, no doubt, have my clinical confreres by the naivete with which these questions have been posed, with the apparent expectation that such answers can be readily provided. It is almost as if an assumption has been made that because psychology is the science (or art) of understanding the mind (as the term is popularly conceived) the psychologist is readily capable of fathoming the complexities underlying the manifestations of brain dysfunction. While we may not actually say so, we imply that our psychometric skills are vastly superior to the neurologist's rubber hammer, and we have in the main, managed to convince neurologists this is so. There is, in our culture, a healthy respect for quantifiable factors. Our tests of perceptual-motor skills, our tests of intellectual function, our other esoteric tests of this and that have convinced a good many people (including sometimes ourselves) that we have the Rosetta Stone which will decipher the secrets of brain dysfunction.

As psychologists, we, on the other hand, are equally impressed by the neurologist's extensive knowledge of the brain, both physiological and anatomical, and look with considerable awe upon his capability to fathom the neurological mysteries of brain function. Neither of us seems willing to recognize, or at least to admit, that there is a great deal of art involved in the practices of clinical neurology and clinical psychology. There is, somehow, a faint stigma attached to the fact that it is, in its ultimate analysis, the clinician's sensitivity which is intimately involved in the decision process; the tests and examinations provide merely the springboard from which the clinician leaps, sometimes into the deep end, in his attempt to fathom the quirks and quiddities of neurological functioning. The quest for a sound scientific basis upon which to make decisions sometimes leads to a ludicrous situation: the neurologist refers the patient to a psychologist for diagnostic studies, the psychologist uses the neurological findings plus his own studies to form a diagnostic opinion and refers the patient back to the neurologist, who then uses the psychologist's opinion to arrive at his definitive diagnosis. Thus, each uses the other's opinion without recognizing that the resultant diagnostic findings are often heavily dependent upon each other without independent validation from sources outside the system. This is, perhaps, a caricature of the true process but it does contain, as Pooh-Bah says in the Mikado ". . . enough historical detail to lend an air of verisimilitude to an otherwise bald and unconvincing narrative."

What I am attempting to point out in this prolegomena to my narrative is that the validity of psychological tests as indices of brain damage is not only a research problem but also, and perhaps more cogently, a clinical problem. It might not be out of place, at this juncture, to remind ourselves of the distinction between an experiment and a piece of research. The distinction is familiar to all of us, but deserves underlining. An experiment, so-called, means traditionally that there are two matched samples, one which we treat and one which we leave untreated. By then comparing these two groups on the relevant dimension in question, we ascertain whether a difference exists. If so, we attribute the difference to our treatment manipulation, all other things being equal. In a research study, on the other hand, we typically have two samples which differ on some variable already present in the experimental sample which is not present in the control sample. We then treat the groups, compare their performances on the relevant dimension and proceed as noted previously. The difference lies in the fact that Nature has, in a sense, already performed the experimental portion of our task for us; i.e., the groups have been differentiated for us prior to our research. Our task, then, is to compare the performances of the group to search out wherein the differences lie. It will have been obvious to the discerning reader what I am driving at; i.e., in our studies of neurological dysfunction, we have examined groups which have been pre-experimentally established; that we have little, if any, knowledge of the parameters determining a particular child's neurological dysfunction. Thus, if differences are observed between groups, it becomes difficult to attribute these differences specifically to neurological dysfunction *per se* because the ultimate source of the differences may lie in other areas.

My purpose in posing this distinction is partly heuristic and partly anticipatory. It is heuristic in that research scientists often blur this distinction and thus obfuscate some of the methodological issues involved; a reminder that it is research and not an experiment that is being conducted may be salutory. It is anticipatory in that some of the paucity of clear-cut research findings among neurologically impaired children (upon which I will touch later) is attributable to an inability to specify the nature of antecedent conditions producing the supposed neurological impairment and subsequent psychological deficit. Having thus perhaps demonstrated I can be abstract, not to say abstruse, let me, in my best organic fashion become more concrete.

UNITARY VERSUS PARTICULARISTIC APPROACHES TO BRAIN DAMAGE

In my discussion of psychological indices of cerebral insult as reflected in the research literature, I shall not attempt to be unitary, i.e., exhaustive. I shall, instead, attempt to be particularistic and selective, rather than taxing your patience with a tedious recapitulation of the state of the art. For those interested in pursuing the field in depth, there are a number of excellent review articles such as those of Meyer (1961), Reitan (1962), and Yates (1954, 1966). My purpose is to consider not the broad field but rather the narrow perspective. Before doing so, however, it will be well to allude to some general research considerations inherent in this particular area of endeavor. The antinomy reflected in the term "unitary" versus "particularistic" seems to be peculiarly a characteristic of research on brain damage. The concept of brain damage seems very often to have meant to most research scientists a single or unitary entity. Therefore, when it constitutes a research group of brain-damaged subjects, a heterogenous variety of neurological impairments might often be subsumed under the rubric of brain-damage and viewed essentially as a homogeneous grouping. In our clinical and theoretical approaches to brain damage, however, we are usually at some pains to distinguish various impairments, such as cognitive, perceptual, or affective components of neurological dysfunction which can be either diffuse or specific, but probably not both. The conceptual distinction between brain damage as a general or unitary entity and brain damage as a particularistic or specific entity is crucial.

On balance, there is considerable evidence that research efforts on neurological dysfunction are becoming increasingly sophisticated. Recent and future research is, and will be, multidimensional in its attack upon problems within the field. That such an approach was necessary has, perhaps, been more evident to the clinician than to the research scientist, since the clinical neurologist and the clinical psychologist were early impressed by the variety of behavioral manifestations which brain damage could elicit. In clinical strategy, as Becker (1963) has pointed out, there are sequential orderings of the diagnostic process which seem to have been mirrored, at least in part, in the evaluation of research on neurological dysfunction. According to him the initial decision is one of presence or absence of brain

damage, and, in order, determination of whether the damage
is diffuse, focal, or multiply focal. Thus, the diagnosis becomes
progressively more refined until a final decision is reached.
It can be noted that research literature on neurological dysfunction somewhat parallels this course, since early research efforts
were directed at ascertaining gross differences between groups.
But present research (Reitan, 1959) has been increasingly refined, and is directed toward more precise localization, both
physically and psychologically, of the effects of brain damage.

Thus, it would appear we are moving toward a general theory
of brain damage which might be analogous to current theories
of intellectual functioning; i.e., we need not concern ourselves
with a dichotomy between generality and specificity, but should
rather consider that brain functions are hierarchically ordered.
Such a view would conclude that the effects of brain damage
are dependent not only upon the fact of cerebral insult itself,
but also upon the location and extent of the cerebral lesion.
Such lesions may also produce widely varying behavioral manifestations, as the research literature abundantly testifies. If this
view is pursued, the apparent diversity of research results may
not reflect so much inadequacies of method, but that each re-
searcher is sampling from a different portion of the population
of brain-damaged individuals. Consequently, the diversities may
reflect the actual complexities of brain dysfunction rather than
reflecting necessarily poor experimental methodology. However,
a review of the literature on brain damage did remind me, as
I attempted to conceptualize brain function, of the quip about
the camel, which was thought to have been a horse designed by
a committee. I was left with something of the same feeling: that
the general topography of brain function was familiar, but that
general agreement was not to be had, and perhaps wisely.

At any rate, I have gone somewhat at length into the foregoing discussion because it is a central issue in the assessment
of the effects of brain damage. If one adopts a position favoring
a unitary conception of brain damage, then one looks for certain
generalized deficits, perhaps overlooking or ignoring specific
effects. If, on the other hand, one adopts a position favoring

a specific or localized concept of the effects of brain damage, then one perhaps overlooks the generalized deficit.

The point, of course, is that research results obtained are largely a function of what one initially has hypothesized in his conceptualization of the problem. The apparently conflicting results may merely reflect that the brain is indeed a complex organ, and that the resultant behavior can be viewed from many different theoretical perspectives. I fear I may have labored this point too long and am reminded you may be thinking somewhat along the same lines as the small boy who, when asked to comment about a book on turtles assigned him by the teacher to review, remarked, "This book tells me more about turtles than I care to know."

EFFECTS OF BRAIN DAMAGE
AND VALIDITY OF PSYCHOLOGICAL TESTS
IN ASSESSING BRAIN DAMAGE

Having brought you thus far, let me finally make bold to commit myself to some comments regarding some effects of brain damage which have bearing upon the focus of this symposium; i.e., brain damage in children. There has been a relative paucity of research literature upon brain damage in children, and the research literature which is available has tended to focus upon the demonstration of differences between these groups and groups of normals. As one reviews this body of literature, one is tempted to sympathize partly with William James' observation that much of our experimental psychology is an elaboration of the obvious. However, my concern is principally that these obtained differences have not been systematically related to antecendent conditions such as locus of the lesion, type of lesion, acuteness or chronicity of the lesion. Without such establishing of the parameters of the brain damage, the utility and generalizability of such findings is limited.

In what follows, I have attempted to focus upon two major areas: *cognitive deficit,* and *perceptual deficit.* I have not attempted to consider the affective deficits which may accompany brain damage. I would classify hyperactivity, lability, and impulsivity under the broad heading of affective deficits (although they certainly have both cognitive and perceptual components) because it is my reasonably firm conviction that such deficits are learned behavior subsequent to the brain trauma and are not a necessary concomitant of brain damage *per se*. This position is partly gained from clinical experience, but also has some roots in the empirical findings of Bijou (1965) as well as others. These findings suggest, *inter alia,* that hyperactivity can be brought quite adequately under operant control indicating that hyperactivity is not "driven" by some brain dysfunction but is, rather, reinforced by environmental circumstance. I shall not digress to pursue this further, except to indicate that it is an area where considerable adjustments in our thinking may be necessary.

To return to the main thrust of my presentation, let me note Hebb's (1949) general discussion of the components of intelligence and attempt to weave it into our discussion in such a manner as to provide an organizing theme for subsequent discussion. It will be recalled that Hebb (1949) has argued for recognition of two components of intelligence. One kind, Intelligence A, has to do with the potential for dealing effectively with both perceptual and conceptual functions, and refers mainly to what might be termed native endowment. Intelligence B refers to those perceptual and conceptual functions found in normal brain function after neurological development has taken place. Thus, Intelligence A represents potential for achievement, while Intelligence B represents past acquisitions. It can be seen that brain damage can affect both kinds of intelligence, but that the effects of such brain damage are likely to be more disorganizing when Intelligence A is affected. It is apparent, of course, that children are more likely to be affected with respect to Intelligence A because they will not have had the opportunity to develop extensive repertoires of Intelligence B.

In this connection, it might be well to note Hunt's very cogent discussion of the effects of various kinds of experiences upon the development of intelligence (1961). In his discussion, Hunt notes there seem to be two major aspects of the brain. One of these is concerned with sensory inputs and the other seems to be concerned with more complex functions which Hunt terms "behavioral strategies"; i.e., higher order behavior influencing thought, language, and so forth. Hunt agrees it is in the latter capacity, that of behavioral strategy, where early experiences have their most salient effects. That is to say, it can be hypothesized that early experiences in the form of various kinds of deprivations have their most central effect by hindering the acquisition of later, more complex, behaviors. It is tempting to extrapolate this to the general area of brain damage in the child because a good deal of research (Strauss and Lehtinen, 1950; Hebb, 1949) supports the notion that damage to the immature brain has considerably more impact on later functioning, particularly cognitive functioning, than does similar damage to the mature brain.

However, it is well to note that such a position is not without its disputants. In particular, Graham et al. (1961, 1962, 1963) note that posing the question in this manner may not be the most meaningful way to consider the problem. It is argued that the question of interest should be whether brain damage produces a similar pattern of impairment in children as it does in adults. If not, what are the differential characteristics produced by such damage in the child? Thus, while it has generally been stated that brain damage in adults produces greater impairment in perceptual-motor and conceptual performance, with less impairment in vocabulary, it is not evident from present research that such a pattern is found in the child. What does seem to have had considerable currency, however, is the impression that the brain-injured child manifests a syndrome of hyperactivity, distractibility, and impulsivity attributed to the brain damage. Addressing themselves to this question, Graham et al. (1963) found that brain-damaged preschool children were significantly inferior in their test performances in perceptual, conceptual, and vocabulary tasks, but not on personality measures. Further, it was noted that the differential pattern of impairment seen in adults, i.e., limited impairment in vocabulary and greater impairment in perceptual-motor and conceptual performances, was not obesrved, but that there was a generalized decrement in all areas. Such a finding lends support to the previous observation that early brain damage may lead to more pronounced general effects than does late brain damage, which may be more selective in its effects.

Graham *et al.* (1963) also marshal evidence to suggest there are differences in the effects of brain damage which are dependent upon the age of the individual and the time at which the damage occurs. At first blush, to argue that there is a generalized damage as well as specific damage may seem inconsistent. What is implied, possibly, is that early damage may produce more generalized deficits, whereas later damage may tend to produce specific deficits. Such a position is consistent with increased localization of function with development. It points up the fact that any discussion of brain damage must also necessarily concern itself with questions of localization of the damage itself, and of the concomitant functions involved. One further finding of interest, before summarizing what has been presented here, was that vocabulary functions seemed to be impaired inversely with age at the time of damage, as opposed to perceptual-motor functions which seemed to be impaired directly with age. Thus, early damage would affect vocabulary relatively greatly, but would not affect perceptual-motor functions markedly; late damage would affect perceptual-motor functions greatly, but would not affect vocabulary functions greatly.

Let us now examine what we have developed, to see what can be gleaned from these findings. We are again confronted with the issue of "unitary" versus "particularistic" viewpoints, as well as the question of localization of the brain damage. In addition, there is the question of the developmental stage at which brain damage has occurred. The Graham *et al.* (1962, 1963) studies were chosen deliberately because they represent a reasonable approach to the problem, an approach implying that damage may be either unitary or particularistic, depending upon the developmental stage of the individual. What has been overlooked, of course, is the question of localization of the lesion, a factor which could have contributed significantly to differential findings. I would argue, however, that in a sample of young children the question of localization of damage may not be as crucial as in the older child or adult. The most salient findings would seem to be:

1) Young brain-damaged children manifest a generalized cognitive and perceptual deficit. 2) Young brain-damaged children do *not* manifest the differential pattern of impairment often observed in adult brain-damaged individuals. 3) The syndrome of hyperactivity, impulsivity, and distractibility considered to be a hallmark of brain damage in children is, perhaps, not a generally distinguishing characteristic of such children.

I would like to conclude this section with the observation that while cognitive deficits are probably a common concomitant of brain damage, they do not account for all of the variance. Such cognitive deficits are likely to be related to the time at which brain damage occurs in the developing individual. All other things being equal, I would argue that early cerebral insult produces generalized cognitive deficits by producing deficits in the capacity for the acquisition and manipulation of new learning skills. While it may affect perceptual-motor functions, it does so only as a generalized factor, and not necessarily as a specific decrement in such skills. I would also note, parenthetically, that clinical experience with retarded children has impressed me much more with cognitive deficits than with perceptual deficits.

Having thus dealt with cognitive deficits, and perhaps having revealed some of my own, let me turn to the area of perceptual deficits in the child and, in particular, the retarded child. In this area I must render a Scottish verdict: i.e., not proven. In reviewing the research literature, it is evident the general burden of the evidence is inconclusive with respect to the question of perceptual deficit in the retardate. It is particularly difficult to tease out the effect of brain damage *per se,* and it is doubly difficult to assign the proper portion to perceptual deficit in and of itself. For example, Gallagher (1957) in a carefully controlled study of brain-damaged and nonbrain-damaged retardates, was unable to demonstrate substantial differences between these groups. Similarly, a study by Ellen Friedman and myself (1963) was unable to elicit differences between such groups.

The thrust of such studies is that perceptual difficulties assignable to brain damage ought to be observable in such groups if generalized perceptual deficits are present. It is recognized such studies do not direct themselves to the question of whether these differences exist between normals and retardates. In general, such differences do exist. However, if one takes cognizance of the fact of differing mental ages (or developmental status) it is questionable whether such differences are attributable to perceptual deficit, mental age, or low ability level. All of the foregoing interact to produce various deficits, and it seems reasonable to question whether such deficits are entirely attributable to brain damage *per se*. Thus, it is questionable whether the problem of establishing definitive indices of perceptual deficit in the retardate has been resolved. Admittedly, I have not dealt at length with the area of perceptual deficit. This is largely because I have not been impressed, both on clinical and experimental grounds, by the actual incidence of perceptual deficits in the retardate. Rather, I have been impressed by the generalized deficits which the retarded child manifests in many areas of his functioning. This latter observation leads me to the conclusion of my presentation.

I would like to conclude by observing that the discriminative validity of psychological tests may be quite adequate for differentiating between normals and retardates with respect to brain damage; the question, however, is the utility of such information. Simply to state that a difference exists is not very useful. We are interested, rather, in the specifics of the manner and degree in which such differences exist, and are further interested in use of such information in a clinically valid and psychologically productive fashion. In conclusion, we may not need further research on brain damage in the retardate, but do need more adequate integration of existing research information with clinical practice.

REFERENCES

1. BIJOU, S. W.: Personal communication, 1965.
2. FRIEDMAN, E., AND BARCLAY, A.: The discriminative validity of certain

psychological tests as indices of brain damage in the mentally retarded. *Ment Retard, 1,* 1963.
3. GRAHAM, F. K., ERNHART, C. B., CRAFT, M., AND BERMAN, P. W.:
Brain injury in the preschool child: Some developmental consideration. *Psychol Monogr,* 77:573, 574, 1663.
4. GRAHAM, F. K., ERNHART, C. B., THURSTON, P., AND CRAFT, M.:
Development three years after perinatal anoxia and other potentially
damaging newborn experiences. *Psychol Monogr,* 76:522, 1962.
5. HEBB, D. O.: *The Organization of Behavior: A Neuropsychological
Theory.* New York, John Wiley, 1949.
6. HUNT, J. McV.: *Intelligence and Experience.* New York, Ronald, 1961.
7. MEYER, V. J.: Psychological effects of brain damage. In Eysenck, H. J.
(Ed.): *Handbook of Abnormal Psychology.* New York, Basic Books,
1961, pp. 529-565.
8. REITAN, R. M.: Psychological deficit. *Ann Rev Psychol, 13*:415-444,
1962.
9. REITAN, R. M.: The effects of brain lesions on adaptive abilities in
human beings. Indianapolis, Mimeo, 1949.
10. STRAUSS, A. A., AND LEHTINEN, L. E.: *Psychopathology and Education
of the Brain Injured Child.* New York, Grune and Stratton, 1950.
11. YATES, A. J.: Psychological deficit. *Ann Rev Psychol, 17*:111-144, 1966.
12. YATES, A. J.: The validity of some psychological tests of brain damage.
Psychol Bull, 51:359-379, 1954.

DISCUSSION I

W. THEODORE MAY, PH.D.

Dr. Barclay's presentation is quite deceptive in that he has
dealt with a number of basic issues in the area—almost without
seeming to do so. It might even be suggested a number of the
notions forwarded in the paper will hopefully be extended and
elaborated upon by him at some future date. Since the material
presented by Dr. Barclay was loaded with implied refutations,
hunches, theoretical formulations and integrations of research
findings and clinical experience, some selection of material for
discussion must obviously take place.

Although never quite stating it directly, Dr. Barclay suggests
we have come along far enough, perhaps, in our understanding
of the area of brain damage so that relatively simplistic notions
of Strauss and Lehtinen (1947) essentially an application of
Goldstein's (1939) notions to children may no longer be an
adequate model either for research or clinical application. Birch

(1964) has suggested, in this connection, that the Strauss-Lehtinen theory did not clearly take into account the variables of location, nature of injury, etc. This shortcoming is being recognized quite generally both in research and clinical work. Reitan and his co-workers have, no doubt, played a major role in this development. However, as clinicians, we may be somewhat reluctant to give up models which have been proven useful—up to a point. If, however, there is reluctance to give up models among psychologists, one should expect much the same response among other professionals, such as physicians or educators. Perhaps continued and expanded multidisciplinary research, teaching and clinical collaboration will, to some extent, offset this particular cultural lag. There can be little doubt that a considerable amount of sophistication is evolving among educators and physicians as increased differentiations are being made of suspect brain-damaged children in terms of such notions as minimally brain-damaged and perceptually handicapped. As one experimental psychologist once said in another connection, "It may not be significant, but it's in the right direction."

It is perhaps at this juncture that Dr. Barclay's admonition to the effect that integration of available research knowledge with clinical practice may be said to be well-taken. Yet, at the same time, one cannot necessarily agree with the suggestion that further research on brain damage in the retardate may not be needed. Several areas must be indicated, at least, which appear to be potentially fruitful. First of all, the matter of base rates has never been systematically studied. Gruenberg (1964), for instance, proposes the need for epidemiological studies to elucidate the prevalence of brain damage in different populations. He suggested the figures on the incidence of brain damage may be a reflection of school system referrals rather than actual incidence. This is apparently what happens in studies with the incidence of mental deficiency; the latter increases up until age thirteen, then drops off. Retarded children frequently leave school shortly after age thirteen, but their level of functioning does not require hospitalization. Longitudinal studies of development, such as the National Institute of Neurological Diseases and Blindness project,[1] may be of great potential usefulness, since it is multidisciplinary. One of the early findings of the local project, however, has introduced unexpected variables such as significant differences in means and variances between experienced examiners in the examination of four-year-olds on the Stanford-Binet (Form L-M). At any rate, longitudinal studies must also take into account pre- and postnatal factors, such as prematurity, toxemia and bleeding during pregnancy, as Knobloch and Pasamanick (1959) have pointed out in their respective studies of the continuum of brain damage. The list of probable antecedent conditions could readily be increased by anyone knowledgeable in the area. Well-done multidisciplinary studies at least could also attempt to cope with criterion problems a little more explicitly.

Secondly, although Dr. Barclay suggests Gallagher (1957) did not find substantial differences between brain-damaged and non-brain-damaged retardates, the findings of the study do suggest that differences seem to exist in various parts of language development. Perhaps the systematic research use of such language development tests as the well-standardized Illinois Test of Psycholinguistic Abilities[2] will prove useful—particularly since the I.T.P.A. has sound theoretical underpinnings, and is intended to fill the gap between diagnosis, program planning and evaluating remedial program effectiveness. This type of approach actually fits in quite well with one of Dr. Barclay's basic contentions, namely, that research and clinical findings of both brain-damaged and retarded children indicate at least the presence of generalized cognitive deficits.

One of Dr. Barclay's major suggestions deals with the issues of unitary versus particularistic approaches to brain damage.

---

[1]Collaborative Project on Cerebral Palsy, Mental Retardation and other Neurological and Sensory Disorders of Infancy and Childhood sponsored by the National Institute of Neurological Diseases and Blindness, National Institutes of Health.

---

[2]*The Illinois Test of Psycholinguistic Abilities,* by James J. McCarthy and Samuel A. Kirk, is published by the University of Illinois Institute for Research on Exceptional Children and distributed by the University of Illinois Press.

It is asserted, in part, that ". . . early cerebral insult produces generalized cognitive deficits by producing deficits in the capacity for the acquisition and manipulation of new learning skills . . .", implying these effects will be more general and more pronounced than the more selective effects of later cerebral insult. Thus, early damage will affect vocabulary more severely than perceptual-motor functions, while later damage will show the reverse. This notion seems to be a particularly fruitful one, fits well into developmental theory and has some evidence to substantiate it. Furthermore, it is based on hierarchical notions in concert with prevailing theoretical frameworks in neurology, intelligence testing and some personality theories.

If the observation that the once-classical syndrome of hyperactivity, distractibility and impulsivity in brain damage are learned behaviors turns out to be correct, some of the variability in the reports of the existence of this triad would be understandable. The possible applicability of operant conditioning to the hyperkinetic syndrome does have appeal. However, one finding would not readily fall into this theoretical construct. This kind of hyperkinetic behavior seems to disappear "spontaneously" sometime between the ages of eight or twelve to eighteen (Laufer, 1962; Cromwell *et al.* 1963).

Dr. Barclay has attempted the perennial task of integrating research findings and clinical experience. This is always a difficult job at best. But one cannot help but be stimulated to rethink commonly acceptable theoretical formulations and unconscious assumptions in terms of the viable notions he presents. If that was the major purpose of the paper, he has succeeded admirably.

REFERENCES

BIRCH, H. G.: The problems of "brain damage" in children. In Birch, H. G. (Ed.): *Brain Damage in Children: Biological and Social Aspects.* Batlimore, Williams and Wilkins, 1964.

CROMWELL, R. L., BAUMEISTER, A., AND HAWKINS, W. F.: Research in activity level. In Ellis, N. R. (Ed.): *Handbook of Mental Deficiency.* New York, McGraw-Hill, 1963.

GALLAGHER, J. J.: A comparison of brain injured and non-brain-injured mentally retarded children on several psychological variables. *Monogr Soc Res Child Develop, 22:*(2), 1957.

GOLDSTEIN, K.: *The Organism.* New York, American Book Company, 1939.

GRUENBERG, H. G.: Some epidemiological aspects of congenital brain damage. In Birch, H. G. (Ed): *Brain Damage in Children: Biological and Social Aspects.* Baltimore, Williams and Wilkins, 1964.

KNOBLOCH, H., AND PASAMANICK, B.: Syndrome of minimal cerebral damage in infancy. *J Amer M A, 170:*1384-1387, 1959.

LAUFER, M. W.: Cerebral dysfunction and behavior disorders in adolescents. *Amer J Orthopsychiat, 32*(3):501-506, 1962.

STRAUSS, A. A., AND LEHTINEN, L. E.: *Psychopathology and Education of the Brain Injured Child.* New York, Grune and Stratton, 1947.

V

POVERTY AND THE BRAIN

WALLACE A. KENNEDY, PH.D.

RECENTLY THE AGE-OLD problem involving interaction between heredity and environment, and functional versus organic trends, has taken some interesting twists. Presently, and in the foreseeable future, separating the effects of strictly environmental or strictly genetic components is an impossible task. But understanding the interaction between the two is essential for understanding the growth and development of children. Many alternate views have been defended through the ages.

HISTORICAL VIEW

Aristotle (384-322 B.C.), like most early scientist-philosophers, and perhaps like most men, believed in the overwhelming importance of the father as the provider of the essential aspect of heredity. "What the male contributes to generation is the form and the efficient cause, while the female contributes the material" (*De Generatione Animalium* 1.20.729a.10-11). Jan Swammerdam (1637-1680) formulated the most tenacious theory, the preformation theory, when he realized that sperm cells in semen were alive and postulated, that these cells were the preformed young, with the egg merely providing nourishment. This preformation theory was complicated by the fertilization theory of Regner de Graaf (1641-1673). So the idea developed, and became firmly entrenched, that in woman, man fertilizes an egg for which she provides heat and protection, and the egg hatches when woman bears man's issue.

Not until the late eighteenth century was the preformation theory put to rest. Kaspar Wolff (1733-1794) discovered in the

110

germ cells of chick embryos undifferentiated substances which, after fertilization, developed potential for body organs, legs, and wings. He demonstrated that at critical periods in development, just before and after fertilization, he could make drastic and specific deformities occur at will. His epigenesis theory was a monumental step toward understanding the role of both sexes in the reproduction process.

At about the same time Jean Lamarck (1744-1829) introduced the tenacious theories of the inheritance of acquired characteristics (experience has the power to make modifications in the body which can be transmitted from generation to generation) and the disuse theory (organs not used eventually become less and less pronounced with each generation until they no longer appear). Lamarck's theories form the basis of Jung's concept of the racial unconscious which proposes that little by little over generations, acquired characteristics are cast into the genes and thus transmitted.

> It [the unconscious] holds possibilities which are locked away from the conscious mind, for it has at its disposal all subliminal contents, all those things which have been forgotten or overlooked, as well as the wisdom and experience of uncounted centuries, which are laid down in its archetypal organs [Jung, 1953, p. 114].

Charles Darwin (1809-1822) next presented his natural selection theory which postulated that only those individuals of a species with the best adaptive characteristics survive and reproduce. In this manner the species grew better and better over generations, more able to cope with the environment. August Weismann (1834-1914) distinguished germ plasm, reproductive cells in the body, from somatoplasm, all other cells in the body. And Hugo DeVries (1848-1935) provided us with the concept of mutation: evolution was neither a gradual eroding away of some unused organ nor the gradual development of some desirable adaptive characteristic, but a series of discrete jumps.

But it was Gregor Mendel (1822-1884) who introduced modern genetics. With five bases, he laid the foundation in genetics for the tremendous advances made in the twentieth century.

1. Genes are the transmitting agents of heredity.

2. At maturity an organism has two or each type of gene.
3. When these two are different, one will be dominant and one recessive.
4. In the germ cells, the genes divide such that each new cell has only one of each type.
5. A random union results in genetic variation.

Thomas Hunt Morgan (1866-1945) discovered that genes are carried in the 23 pairs of chromosomes of the cell nucleus like beads on a string, rather than like chips or marble; that is, genes are transported in linked fashion and do not divide merely by chance. Then in 1958, George Beadle and Edward Tatum won the Nobel Prize for Medicine by discovering that DNA (desoxyribonucleic acid) and RNA (ribonucleic acid) are protein molecules which act by regulating definite chemical metabolic reactions. Obviously, then, any change in the genes would affect the chemical balance in the body.

So, modern research has taught us that experience does indeed have the power to make changes passed from one generation to the next, but these are a result only of biochemical experience. Environment definitely can influence heredity, but only through the avenue of body chemistry which affects the organization of DNA and RNA. Over time, then, alternative views have been presented about the differing effects of heredity and environment.

Summary of Historical Views

The first feels that the mother serves merely as an incubator, with little or no interaction between her and her baby. Successful abdominal pregnancies tended to give support to those who believed in a passive, almost independent relationship between mother and child during pregnancy.

A second view holds that the mother can affect her unborn child even by seeing an ugly or frightening sight. Although once pooh-poohed by so-called sophisticated people, this view is closer to the truth than the first one. Modern research has clearly demonstrated that upset mothers produce upset infants. Not only can genetic diseases be transferred from one generation to another, such as Rh-factor problems, hemophilia, Down's syndrome, and sex chromosome and metabolic anomalies, but relatively harmless diseases of the mother during pregnancy can wreak devastating havoc upon the unborn child, maternal rubella (measles) being one of the greatest offenders. Drugs taken by the mother during pregnancy, her smoking habits, especially her diet, all affect the unborn child. Even the mother's emotional state can be transferred to the child by hormone transference through the placenta. Studies of the mother's emotional state during pregnancy and the child's adjustment after birth have uncovered a significant relationship between the mother and child. About the child, Montagu writes:

> He is to all intents and purposes a neurotic infant when he is born—the result of an unsatisfactory fetal environment. In this instance he has not had to wait until childhood for a bad home situation or other cause to make him neurotic. It has been done for him before he has even seen the light of day [1954, p. 19].

A third view follows the theories of Lamarck and Jung and suggests that little by little over many generations characteristics are acquired and transmitted. Such a belief could have grown out of DeVries' mutation theory, if one considers the fact that most mutations are lethal and only a very few adaptive ones survive, or Darwin's theory of the survival of the fittest, for gradually over generations only the most adaptive characteristics would survive. With modern medicine, however, infant mortality rates are growing ever lower and no longer do only the fittest survive to the age of reproduction.

A fourth view holds that little development occurs before birth, when suddenly environmental effects come to bear. This view holds that, in general, we are all born with somewhat equal potential and that environmental stimulation determines the direction and amount of growth.

Clearly, environment has been demonstrated to affect significantly measured intelligence. But research has already indicated that environmental effect begins even before conception, through the health of the parents to be, and certainly is present during pregnancy at all stages, but most particularly during the rapid development of the first trimester. Environmental damage prior to birth may already have made the child unable to use advantageously the best of all environments after birth.

Zigler's two-group approach to mental retardation leads us into a fifth view, the brain-damage point of view, which speaks in terms of some kind of biological potential for normal growth in all; a potential, however, markedly reducible by a developmental or traumatic event occurring during pregnancy or the birth process.

Not all men are created equal in intelligence if one considers the normal distribution of any population and its characteristic bell-shaped curve, with most of the population clustered in the middle, but with some few individuals stretched out above and below the mean. Without ever having heard of "statistics" and "normal distributions," men have always been aware of the genius and the idiot.

> Approached in this way, the familial retardate can be seen as normal, where normal is defined as representing an integral part of the distribution of intelligence that we would expect from the normal manifestations of the genetic pool in our population. . . . Considerable clarity could be brought to the area of mental retardation if we were to do away with the practice of conceptualizing the intelligence distribution as a single continuous normal curve. Perhaps a more appropriate representation is to depict the intelligence of the bulk of the population, including the familial retarded, as a normal distribution having a mean of 100 with lower and upper limits approximately 50 and 150, respectively. Superimposed on this curve would be a second somewhat normal distribution having a mean of approximately 35 and a range from zero to 70. The first curve would represent the polygenic distribution of intelligence; the second would represent all those individuals whose intellectual functioning reflected factors other than the normal polygenic expression, i.e., those retardates for whom there is an identifiable physiological defect [Zigler, 1966, p. 123].

Some psychologists and neurologists have begun to speak with a great deal of certainty, not only about the amount and kind of brain damage, but also about the resulting percentage of deficit. This view, while entirely plausible, suffers from the absence of adequate normative data. What is the incidence of nonclinical lesions in the normal population?

DEPRIVATION AND PHYSICAL ENVIRONMENT

Research has long pointed up a significant relationship between deprivation and the development of potential. Beadle and Tatum first suggested that the gene represents an enzyme molecule similar in action to an industrial computer program which directs the complex milling processes. The gene, however, dictates the complex synthesizing of an enzyme consisting of hundreds of amino acid units arranged end to end in a specific and unique order. A gene mutation, often resulting from a single ionization, may serve not only as an enzyme, but as a catalyst for the production of new enzymes, and thus is analogous to altering an industrial template during the process of milling, a change which would result not simply in the alteration of one unit, but in all the following units in production.

The hereditary link of the gene is insulated from the wear and tear of every-day experience. However, anything which causes massive chemical changes within the body could well alter the template and thus introduce massive changes in the growth pattern of the whole individual. These are not simply complex, massive changes resulting from irradiation-caused mutations, but hormonal changes, and changes to the DNA substance as a result of psychological and physical stress.

Animal research on the effects of malnutrition has indicated the need to take into account the nutritional history of previous generations (Cowley, 1968), because malnutrition affects not only growth and learning, but also behavior. Pasamanick (1946; Knobloch and Pasamanick, 1960) has called attention to the relationship between cultural deprivation and all types of physical abnormalities seemingly related to prenatal and postnatal environmental factors affecting the child. According to Lyle, reading retardation is

> an inherent learning difficulty which includes the learning of speech and even of arithmetical calculation, and which has some ill-

defined and tenuous connections with anomalies of the perinatal and postnatal periods [1970, p. 490].

MALNUTRITION

Recently much research has been expended upon the importance of nutrition in these physical and mental abnormalities and the interrelatedness of malnutrition and deprivation. Clearly, researchers, both laboratory and field, have concluded that the two go hand in hand inseparably.

> Our observations indicate that early malnutrition tends to restrict expression of the genetic potential for development, both physical and psychological. Socio-economic factors also strongly affect mental development and cannot be separated satisfactorily from nutritional influences [Monckeberg, 1968, pp. 276-277].

The emphasis, then, is on the effect of malnutrition and deprivation, and remediation.

Animal Studies

Laboratory study of malnutrition and undernutrition in animals has now very clearly indicated that permanent damage in brain growth, as well as overall physical growth, learning ability, and behavior, follows malnutrition at critical periods. The brain grows rapidly during the first few months of life, and this growth is largely a process of protein synthesis (Monckeberg, 1968; Ogata *et al.*, 1968). Malnutrition in animals not only stunts physical growth, but also reduces subsequent learning ability and memory, and adversely affects behavior (Keppel, 1968). A protein deficiency in the first few weeks of pregnancy results in considerable distortion in brain growth with the higher centers of the brain seeming to receive the major brunt of the deficiency (Venkatachalam and Ramanathan, 1964; Cowley, 1968; Gordon and Deanin, 1968). Stewart and Platt noticed changes in physique and behavior in pigs offered unlimited amounts of low-protein diet. These same changes have been recorded "in human subjects suffering from protein-calorie deficiency" (1968, p. 169).

Permanent and catastrophic changes in essential organs, including the brain, can be achieved by applying stress of various kinds (i.e., diet restriction, infection, drug ingestion, etc.) during critical periods of early prenatal development. These stresses can also operate much later in prenatal and postnatal life to produce a different long-range effect. Permanent reduction in body and brain size are produced in rats by comparatively mild under-nutrition confined to the first three weeks of life. Both the rate and ultimate extent of growth is affected (Dobbing, 1968).

On the other hand, the adult brain is highly resistant to changes in weight, even in the most severe starvation, provided it is able to grow normally to a mature size before the starvation begins. Animal research indicates that the effects of undernutri-tion on the brain depend upon the timing of the undernutrition in relation to the period of fastest brain growth. The first three to five days after birth appear to be uniquely important. Thus, a "carry-over of gestational dietary effects on the mother into these first few days could produce growth inhibition even when the maternal diet had been shifted at birth" (Miller, 1968, p. 231).

> Animals fed only one fourth of a balanced diet or a diet isocaloric with that of normally fed controls but with only a fourth of the normal protein content showed reduced growth without other clinical signs suggestive of malnutrition. This is of course the status of the majority of young children in developing countries. For this reason, the fact that these animals were inactive, demonstrated little interest in their environment, and showed other signs of retarded social development is of more than academic interest. . . . Malnutrition in the early life of experimental animals has a direct effect on sub-sequent function of the central nervous system. . . . As expected, deficiencies induced in the experimental animal soon after birth have more of an effect on learning and behavior than those initiated at the end of normal lactation [Scrimshaw and Gordon, 1968, p. 249].

Human Studies

A high correlation has been demonstrated between maternal nutrition and infant mortality and morbidity (Ebbs *et al.*, 1942; Warkany, 1944, 1947; Burke and Stuart, 1952; Wortis, 1963; Bayley, 1965; Knobloch and Pasamanick, 1966; Pasamanick and Knobloch, 1966).

Retardation of physical growth and development due to nutritional deficiency is widespread and clearly recognized in developing countries; it is all too frequent in our own urban slums and rural pockets of poverty. That malnutrition also may influence mental development, learning, and behavior lifts this concern to a wholly new level of world importance [Johnson, 1968, p. 2].

Any study of causal relationship between malnutrition and its consequences in infants and young children must consider at least three sets of associated factors. The first is availability of nutrients to the body tissues—the quality and quantity of food ingested by the child. The second set involves features of health and disease which directly or indirectly affect dietary intake and nutritional status, of which infections appear to play a major role. The third set of factors is of a general social character, including such influences as social and economic status, educational background of parents, and patterns of child care.

Because of the intimate association between nutrition and income level in almost all societies, malnourished persons as well as children previously at nutritional risk tend to cluster heavily in the underprivileged segments of a population. Such segments differ from the remainder not only in increased exposure to nutritional stresses but also in many other variables. They tend to have poorer housing, lower levels of formal education, higher incidence of infectious disease, greater attachment to outmoded patterns of child care, obsolete concepts of causes of health and disease, and in general they live in circumstances less conducive to development of technologic and educational competence. Moreover, the effects of these circumstances may continue from one generation to another and suggest a familial or hereditary process. . . .

Because of these facts and associations, it is inevitable that any after effects in physical or mental growth will be associated with social status. There has been a tendency to view these relations in a circular fashion and to conclude that social status of itself accounts for disturbed developmental outcomes. This unfortunately substitutes a truism for an analysis. Given the associations between low social standing and undesirable physical and mental outcomes, the task of analysis is to tease out the effective variables that mediate these outcomes. Clearly, social class as such does not determine stature. Rather, individuals are stunted when their social positions provide a poor general environment in such terms as nutrition, infection, habits, and housing, which influence adversely the biological processes involved in growth. Similarly, mental growth is modified to the degree that conditions of life associated with low social position act to modify directly the growth and differentiation of the central nervous system, and indirectly the opportunities and motives to learn from experience. . . .

The data lead to a prediction that the shorter children, whose height is a reflection of earlier and sometimes continuing malnutrition, risk school failure stemming from an incapacity to master primary school subjects. If this prediction is substantiated, as preliminary field observation suggests, early malnutrition from either primary or secondary sources may be the starting point of a developmental path characterized by neurointegrative inadequacy, school failure, and subsequent subnormal adaptive functioning [Cravioto and De Licardie, 1968, pp. 253, 267].

PREMATURITY

Although adequate comparisons are difficult, we know that "premature infants have two to three times as many physical defects, 50 per cent more illnesses, and a significantly higher number of neurological impairments" (Kennedy, 1971, p. 36). Braine *et al.* (1966) found a significant relationship between degree of impairment and degree of prematurity. And the mother's diet, smoking, and economic status are all related to the maturity or prematurity of her infant. Simpson (1957) and Frazier *et al.* (1961) found twice as high an incidence of prematurity in infants of cigarette-smoking mothers. Corah *et al.* (1965) found prematurely born children significantly impaired in cognitive and perceptual motor tests irrespective of whether they had suffered anoxia.

Because of the difficulty in always correctly judging fetal age, any infant weighing less than five and a half pounds at birth is usually considered premature. Note, however, that prematurity per se does not necessarily interfere to the slightest degree in normal brain development, but that small brain development, in relationship to fetal age, resulting from a defective placenta, fetal incompatibility, or inadequate blood supply, has long-term detrimental effects.

Equally important, the fetus is in a position of much greater invulnerability to nutritional deficiency than is the newborn infant, because the fetus can indeed obtain nourishment through his parasitic relationship to the mother. Malnutrition, then, during the prenatal period results not so much from malnourishment of the mother as from the failure of the placenta to deliver proper amounts of nourishment. A fetus, then, is relatively immune to the poor nutrition of the mother, provided that at birth he is nursed by a well-fed foster mother.

On the other hand, if a maternal nutritional deficiency exists during the prenatal period and continues during the early post-natal period, malnutrition is very apt to have a profound effect upon the development of the brain, the physical growth, learning ability, and behavior of the young child. This is so for two reasons. First, a fixed quantity of nutrition is produced through the mother's milk; if she is suffering from severe malnutrition, her milk suffers quantitatively and qualitatively. Second, the child's balance in nutrition is so critical that even a short period of three to five days of malnutrition has a serious effect.

Gruenwald makes the important point that true prematures catch up in height and weight, "while growth-retarded fetuses [underweight-for-age] remain below the third percentile for height and weight. In other words, they are growth-retarded for a long period of time, perhaps permanently," despite a subsequently improved nutrition (1968, p. 305).

INFECTIOUS DISEASES

The relationship between infectious diseases and poverty is obvious. And, "both in the United States and in less well developed areas, infections account for a significant proportion of permanent neuronal damage" (Eichenwald, 1968, p. 435). Syphilis, thyroid disorders, subclinical or prediabetes, as well as diabetes, heart disease, even influenza and mumps contracted by the mother during pregnancy, all produce deleterious effects upon the unborn fetus. As research on maternal rubella has become increasingly more sophisticated, increasingly greater adverse effects have been demonstrated on the unborn child (Dunphy, 1945; Pasamanick, 1946; Rhodes, 1961; Emery, 1968). Not only does the child have a 60 per cent chance of being abnormal in some way through deafness, eye defects, and heart disease, but his mental functioning is impaired.

STIMULATION

Frankova reported that "a reduced caloric intake in the early stages of development results in decreased spontaneous activity of adult rats. The effect may be modified appreciably by stimulation" (1968, p. 321). The studies of Hein (1968) and Altman (1968) demonstrated the power of purely experiential factors without any overt biochemical or anatomical intervention, in influencing development and maturation. They are examples of the role that social environmental experiences alone can play in the development process.

> In animal experiments sensory deprivation interferes with both morphological and functional development of the central nervous system. In children, lack of stimulation and attention impairs normal mental development and alters social behavior. . . . These conclusions precisely parallel those established for experimental malnutrition in animals and claimed for human populations [Scrimshaw and Gordon, 1968, p. 384].

Plenty of evidence is available to indicate that lack of perceptual stimulation in the first few weeks after birth may well profoundly affect the development of the functional relationships within the central nervous system. Stimulation has been found to increase the infant's responsiveness and interest in his external environment (Schaffer and Emerson, 1964a,b; White and Castle, 1964; Moss, 1970). Yarrow (1963) reported that the amount and quality of maternal stimulation greatly influenced the infant's development during the first six months, based on IQ scores. Fantz (1966) and Korner and Grobstein (1966) suggest that crib stimulation, through multiple media, sound, light, vibration, plus constant perceptual contrast, and maternal soothing of the neonate have a marked effect upon the development of children's conceptual strength.

A definitive study on the effects of poor postnatal nutrition on intelligence is extraordinarily difficult due to the confounding of nutritional and other environmental deficiencies; that is, children, who are born of malnourished mothers and who are malnourished themselves during the first few weeks of life, are also children who are exposed to extremely primitive environments. Only in cases of sudden famine in an ordinarily enriched society can definitive field studies be done. Yet, the field studies conducted around the world, in spite of their shortcomings, all support the findings with experimental animals that early malnutrition and undernutrition can definitely interfere with learning and behavior.

Repeated demonstrations have been made of the similarity in effect between prenatal and early postnatal malnutrition and early sensory deprivation on learning and behavior of children—that early malnutrition and early sensory deprivation, or lack of psychological and social stimuli, can produce the same deleterious effects. The fact that these are often tandem influences creates a crushing deficit in the early learning of the culturally deprived child.

DEPRIVATION AND NEUROLOGICAL DEFICIT

Genetic variation is inherent in any biological process. Within limits determined by the genotype, structure and function are subject to modification by environmental influences to give a wide range of phenotypes and responses of the central nervous system to stimuli [Scrimshaw and Gordon, 1968, p. 164].

Over and over again one sees the relationship between the general health of infants, as well as their neurological growth, and environmental deprivation, especially dietary and prenatal-care deprivation during the prenatal period. Because, then, of the multitude of adverse factors associated with the prenatal and early postnatal development of culturally deprived infants, these children have a higher probability of neurological deficit than the average child.

In a normative study of 1,800 children in the southeast, the greatest majority of whom fell into the lowest socioeconomic levels, Kennedy, Van De Riet, and White (1963) found that these children obtained uniformly low scores on achievement and intellectual measurements, and that these scores correlated positively with socioeconomic level. The mean Stanford-Binet IQ for this normative sample of black children, studied on a stratified, random basis from urban, rural, and metropolitan elementary schools, was 80, with a proportional deficit demonstrated on the

California Achievement Test. Motor skills, motor development, and visual motor development, particularly as measured by the Goodenough Draw-A-Man Test's perception of human form, were also positively related to socioeconomic level.

Two obvious interpretations can be made of the 20-point mean difference between this low socioeconomic group and the middle-class population of the country upon which the 1960 Binet was standardized. The first considers an intelligence test developed and standardized for one population unsuitable for another population and therefore invalid. Thus, the deficit in IQ obtained for the culturally deprived group is simply a function of the unsuitability of the test for this population, since intelligence may be defined as the amount of cultural assimilation an individual child has managed. To measure this cultural assimiliation, one has to measure the variables within the culture of this child. This line of reasoning concludes that the solution to the obtained deficit would be in the creation of a new intelligence test suitable for making predictions regarding this cultural minority's adaptation to its environment. This seems an unrealistic interpretation toward the end of the twentieth century in the United States.

A second broader and more realistic interpretation of this deficit is that it is a real and highly significant one. The factors sampled by this test are indeed significant in predicting adaptation to the American culture, most particularly to the American middle-class educational system as a whole, and most strikingly at the upper grade levels. Thus it would be predicted that children who score poorly on major intelligence and achievement tests will be at a severe disadvantage throughout their lives in attempting to adjust to the middle-class domination of the schools and upper end of the employment continuum. This interpretation holds that the development of any artificial tests applied to black children only, or to deprived children only, would lose all relevance if used outside the deprived area. Good adjustment or bad adjustment to a deprived area is probably of little significance when considered in light of the goals of American democracy.

Unfortunately, unless new and radically different educational methods are developed, the gloomy prediction stands. One-fifth of the 1960 sample, 312 of the 360 children, were located and retested five years later (Kennedy, 1969). The IQ remained substantially the same for this group of the sample. In 1960, the mean IQ was 79.2; in 1965, 79.4. Obviously, this was a non-significant change. The standard deviation increased from 12.6 in 1960 to 14.3 in 1965, with the range in scores also increasing slightly. Although the IQ's tended to remain constant across grade levels, as had been observed in 1960, there was the obvious decline in IQ associated with chronological age.

This finding (illustrated in Tables I and II [Kennedy, 1969, p. 20, Table 3]) confirms the hypothesis projected by Schaefer in 1965, that the sampling method of representing grades instead of chronological age produced a negative correlation of mean IQ with age. Thus, because of promotional policies in school, a greater percentage of duller children were found in the upper age range. This was a sampling artifact rather than any trend, since the IQ's of the individual children did not decrease over an age span. The hypothesis was further confirmed since the mean IQ did not decrease over the four-year span.

TABLE I

STANFORD-BINET IQ MEANS AND STANDARD DEVIATIONS BY GRADE

Grade	N	1960 Mean	S.D.	N	1965 Mean	S.D.
1	52	81.2	9.7			
2	52	77.8	13.5			
3	53	81.4	14.3			
4	53	76.9	12.5	16	76.7	9.3
5	50	78.9	12.9	46	85.3	15.0
6	52	79.1	13.6	56	81.0	14.0
7				56	81.7	14.4
8				44	75.3	14.6
9				56	75.8	16.0
10				38	77.7	13.9
Total	312	79.2	12.6	312	79.4	14.3

This entire population was found to have difficulty on visual motor tasks. Thus the general belief that black children are skilled in motor tasks with verbalization being their only intellectual problem was not confirmed. The Stanford-Binet Form

TABLE II

STANFORD-BINET IQ MEANS AND STANDARD DEVIATIONS
BY CHRONOLOGICAL AGE

C.A.	N	1960 Mean	S.D.	N	1965 Mean	S.D.
5	12	86.8	7.6			
6	47	83.2	9.4			
7	41	81.6	13.3			
8	53	79.7	12.5			
9	45	77.5	13.0			
10	48	79.8	15.3	40	90.0	11.3
11	43	76.9	12.4	39	84.1	11.6
12	12	69.9	7.1	50	85.6	13.9
13	7	67.1	8.1	44	77.3	10.5
14	4	63.3	9.0	54	76.3	15.1
15				48	75.0	17.0
16				26	68.8	13.0
17				7	64.6	9.2
18				3	67.7	16.1
19				1	74.0	0.0
Total	312	79.2	12.6	312	79.4	14.3

L-M and the Goodenough Draw-a-Man Test both indicated a high frequency of organic signs and a nearly normal distribution of these signs. The frequency was too high and the distribution too symmetrical for the organic signs to be the result of brain lesions. It is significant, however, that the poor medical care and general lack of nutrition for the pregnant mother, and continuing poor nutrition and lack of stimulation for the child, indicate a distinct possibility that central nervous system damage would be more likely to occur in this population. Yet, we must remember that tests of the central nervous system all depend to a great extent on early experience and early practice; a small amount of prepractice on a related task can make improvements in the Bender-Gestalt performance of deprived children (Kaspar and Schulman, 1964).

And, in considering the use of psychological tests for the diagnosis of brain damage, the attitude of the subject toward the examiner has been suggested as having a strong effect on the motivation and set during the testing. But research at FSU makes the author contend that the examiner effect is minimal at the school-age level (Kennedy and Willcutt, 1964; Tiber and Kennedy,

1964; Kennedy and Vega, 1965), although Katz (1964 seems to think not.

Also, intrinsic motivation has been suggested as a problem, wherein the deprived child may approach the testing situation with a lower level of motivation than the middle-class child; that is, the tests themselves do not have the interest for lower-class children as they do for middle-class children. Tiber and Kennedy, however, found that manipulating the motivation on intelligence tests by various incentive changes did not reveal any significant effects.

DEPRIVATION AND EXPERIENCE

Culturally deprived children, reared in homes without crayons, pencils, drawing boards, blackboards and games, suffer a deficit in their perceptual ability, a deficit which may be modifiable, but which closely resembles central nervous system damage. This was brought out clearly in the Farmville, Virginia, project, where we tested children who had been out of school for four years. They, as well as those who had never gone to school, were not only unable to make the letters of the alphabet, but were literally unable to hold pencils in their hands.

Hess and Shipman (1965a,b) and Olim, Hess, and Shipman (1967) showed, in a convincing demonstration, how poorly mothers of low socioeconomic status communicate instructions to their children. Hess gave the mothers nonverbal instructions on playing a game, which they were then required to teach verbally to their children. The low socioeconomic mothers were unable to explain the game at all unless allowed to demonstrate.

Thus, we must be extremely careful in conceptualizing what is physical and what is learned. Allowances must be made for the fact that good animal research indicates that stimulus deprivation and experience deprivation may lead to a permanent deficit in visual motor ability unrelated to actual damage to the central nervous system. In speaking of the effects of cultural deprivation upon the developing intellect, J. McV. Hunt emphasizes the probable seriousness of continued deprivation in the necessary environmental stimulation for healthy maturation and development.

The longer these conditions continue, the more likely the effects are to be lasting. . . . Tadpoles immobilized with chlorotone for 8 days are not greatly hampered in the development of their swimming patterns, but immobilization for 13 days leaves their swimming patterns permanently impaired; chicks kept in darkness for as many as 5 days show no apparent defects in their pecking responses, but keeping them in darkness for 8 or more days results in chicks which never learn to peck at all [1964, p. 89].

It would seem important, then, before generating hypotheses about the existence of obscure lesions, or that these lesions are relevant, that one should first take into account the possibility that the child has not had adequate experience with the types of stimuli being presented.

SUMMARY

So, we have outlined two significant, interrelated factors relating central nervous system functioning and cultural deprivation. First, the central nervous system apparently encompasses both organic and functional aspects, and second, cultural deprivation plays a significant role in each of these.

Without adequate obstetrical care, nutrition, and disease prevention, the brain can be damaged structurally to the point where its function is significantly below its biological capacity—poverty minority groups suffer from the poorest nutritional, medical, and public health care imaginable.

Without adequate early perceptual, conceptual, and language stimulation, the internal functional organization of the brain does not seem to develop to its full potential—the first few months and years of life seem the most critical. The walls of the ghetto insulate the deprived child from this essential external stimulation to an alarming and critical degree.

Surely there can be no question that cultural deprivation plays a key role in the functioning of the central nervous system!

REFERENCES

ALTMAN, JOSEPH: Effects of early experience on brain morphology. In Scrimshaw and Gordon: *Malnutrition, Learning and Behavior*, Cambridge, The M.I.T. Press, 1968, pp. 332-346.

BAYLEY, NANCY: Comparisons of mental and motor test scores for ages 1-15 months by sex, birth order, race, geographic location, and education of parents. *Child Dev, 36:*379-411, 1965.

BRAINE, MARTIN D. S., HEIMER, CARYL B., WORTIS, HELEN, AND FREEDMAN, ALFRED M.: Factors associated with impairment of the early development of prematures. *Monogr Soc Res Child Dev, 31(4) (No. 106)*, 1966.

BURKE, B. S., AND STUART, H. C.: Nutritional requirements during pregnancy and lactation. In *Handbook of Nutrition*, 2d ed. London, H. K. Lewis & Co., 1952.

CHOW, BACON F.: Short comment. In Scrimshaw and Gordon: *Malnutrition, Learning and Behavior*, Cambridge, The M.I.T. Press, 1968, pp. 228-229.

CORAH, NORMAN L., ANTHONY, E. J., PAINTER, P., STERN, JOHN A., AND THURSTONE, D.: Effects of perinatal anoxia after seven years. *Psychol Monogr, 79(3) (No. 596)*, 1965.

COWLEY, JOHN J.: Time, place, and nutrition: some observations from animal studies. In Scrimshaw and Gordon: *Malnutrition, Learning and Behavior*, Cambridge, The M.I.T. Press, 1968, pp. 218-227.

CRAVIOTO, JOAQUIN, AND DE LICARDIE, ELSA R.: Intersensory development of school-age children. In Scrimshaw and Gordon: *Malnutrition, Learning and Behavior*, Cambridge, The M.I.T. Press, 1968, pp. 252-268.

DOBBING, JOHN: The influence of nutrition on the development and myelination of the brain. *Proceedings of the Royal Society, Biology, 159, 503,* 1964.

DOBBING, JOHN: Effects of experimental undernutrition on development of the nervous system. In Scrimshaw and Gordon: *Malnutrition, Learning and Behavior*, Cambridge, The M.I.T. Press, 1968, pp. 181-202.

DUNPHY, E. B.: Medical progress: ophthalmology. *N Engl J Med, 232:*675-682, 1945.

EBBS, J. H., BROWN, A., TISDALL, F. F., MOYLE, W. J., AND BELL, M.: The influence of improved prenatal nutrition upon the infant. *Can Med Assoc J, 46:*6-8, 1942.

EICHENWALD, HEINZ F.: Prenatal and postnatal infectious diseases affecting the central nervous system. In Scrimshaw and Gordon: *Malnutrition, Learning and Behavior*, Cambridge, The M.I.T. Press, 1968, pp. 426-437.

EMERY, ALAN, E. H.: *Heredity, Disease, and Man: Genetics in Medicine.* Berkeley, University of California Press, 1968.

FANTZ, ROBERT L.: The crucial early influence: mother love or environmental stimulation? *Am J Orthopsychiatry, 36:*330-331, 1966 (Abstract).

FRANKOVA, SLAVKA: Nutritional and psychological factors in the development of spontaneous behavior in the rat. In Scrimshaw and Gordon: *Malnutrition, Learning and Behavior*, Cambridge, The M.I.T. Press, 1968, pp. 312-322.

FRAZIER, TODD M., DAVIS, GEORGE H., GOLDSTEIN, HYMAN, AND GOLDBERG, IRVING D.: Cigarette smoking and prematurity: a prospective study. *Am J Obstet Gyn, 81*:988-996, 1961.

somes: a proposal on the protein nutrition of the synapse. In Scrimshaw GORDON, MALCOLM W., AND DEANIN, GRACE G.: Mitochondria and lyso- and Gordon: *Malnutrition, Learning and Behavior,* Cambridge, The M.I.T. Press, 1968, pp. 136-150.

GRUENWALD, PETER: Short comment. In Scrimshaw and Gordon: *Malnutrition, Learning and Behavior,* Cambridge, The M.I.T. Press, 1968, pp. 304-307.

HEIN, ALAN: Labile sensorimotor coordination. In *Malnutrition, Learning and Behavior,* by Scrimshaw and Gordon: Cambridge, The M.I.T. Press, 1968, pp. 327-332.

HESS, ROBERT D., AND SHIPMAN, VIRGINIA C.: Early blocks to children's learning. *Children, 12*:189-194, 1965a.

HESS, ROBERT D., AND SHIPMAN, VIRGINIA C.: Early experience and the socialization of cognitive modes in children. *Child Dev, 36*:869-886, 1965b.

HUNT, J. McVICKERS: How children develop intellectually. *Children, 11*:83-91, 1964.

JOHNSON, HOWARD W.: *Society, nutrition, and research.* In Scrimshaw and Gordon: *Malnutrition, Learning and Behavior,* Cambridge, The M.I.T. Press, 1968, pp. 2-4.

JUNG, CARL G.: *Two Essays on Analytical Psychology.* Vol. 7 of *Collected Works.* Edited by Herbert Read, Michael Fordham, and Gerhard Adler. Translated by R. F. C. Hall. New York, Pantheon Press, 1953.

KASPAR, JOSEPH C., AND SCHULMAN, J. L.: The explication and solution of a specific error in copying diamonds. *J Exp Child Psychol, 1*:311-315, 1964.

KATZ, I.: Review of evidence relating to the effects of desegregation on the intellectual performance of Negroes. *Am Psychol, 19*:381-399, 1964.

KENNEDY, WALLACE A.: A follow-up normative study of Negro intelligence and achievement. *Monogr Soc Res Child Dev, 34(2), (No. 126),* 1969.

KENNEDY, WALLACE A.: *Child Psychology.* Englewood Cliffs, Prentice-Hall, 1971.

KENNEDY, WALLACE A., VAN DE RIET, VERNON, AND WHITE, JAMES C., JR.: A normative sample of intelligence and achievement of Negro elementary school children in the southeastern United States. *Monogr Soc Res Child Dev, 28(6), No. 90,* 1963.

KENNEDY, WALLACE A., AND VEGA, MANUEL: Negro children's performance on a discrimination task as a function of examiner race and verbal incentive. *J Per Soc Psychol, 2*:839-843, 1965.

KENNEDY, WALLACE A., AND WILLCUTT, HERMAN C.: Praise and blame as incentives. *Psychol Bull, 62*:323-332, 1964.

KEPPEL, FRANCIS: Food for thought. In Scrimshaw and Gordon: *Malnutrition, Learning and Behavior*, Cambridge, The M.I.T. Press, 1968, pp. 4-9.

KNOBLOCH, HILDA, AND PASAMANICK, BENJAMIN: Environmental factors affecting human development before and after birth. *Pediatrics, 26:*210-218, 1960.

KNOBLOCH, HILDA, AND PASAMANICK, BENJAMIN: Prospective studies of the epidemiology of reproductive casualty: methods, findings, and some implications. *Merrill-Palmer Quarterly of Behavior and Development, 12:*27-43, 1966.

KORNER, ANNELIESE F., AND GROBSTEIN, ROSE: Visual alertness as related to soothing in neonates: implications for maternal stimulation and early deprivation. *Child Dev, 37:*867-876, 1966.

LEVINE, SEYMOUR: Psychophysiological effects of infantile stimulation. In *Roots of Behavior: Genetics, Instinct, and Socialization in Animal Behavior*. Edited by E. Bliss. New York, Hoeber Medical Book, Harper & Bros., 1962.

LYLE, J. G.: Certain antenatal, perinatal, and developmental variables and reading retardation in middle-class boys. *Child Dev, 41:*481-491, 1970.

MILLER, SANFORD A.: Short comment. In *Malnutrition, Learning and Behavior*, by Scrimshaw and Gordon, Cambridge, The M.I.T. Press, 1968, pp. 229-232.

MONCKEBERG, FERNANDO: Effect of early marasmic malnutrition on subsequent physical and psychological development. In Scrimshaw and Gordon: *Malnutrition, Learning and Behavior*, Cambridge, The M.I.T. Press, 1968, pp. 269-278.

MONTAGU, M. F. ASHLEY: Constitutional and prenatal factors in infant and child health. In *Readings in Child Dev*, Edited by William E. Martin and Celia Burns Stendler. New York, Harcourt, Brace, 1954, pp. 15-29.

MOSS, HOWARD A.: Early environmental effects: mother-child relations. Chapter 1 in *Perspectives in Child Psychology: Research and Review*. Edited by Thomas D. Spencer and Norman Kass. New York, McGraw-Hill, 1970, pp. 3-34.

OGATA, K., KIDO, H., ABE, S., FURUSAWA, Y., AND SATAKE, M.: Activity of protein synthesis of the brain of protein-deficient rats. In Scrimshaw and Gordon: *Malnutrition, Learning and Behavior*, Cambridge, The M.I.T. Press, 1968, pp. 131-135.

OLIM, ELLIS, G., HESS, ROBERT D., AND SHIPMAN, VIRGINIA C.: Role of mothers' language styles in mediating their preschool children's cognitive development. *School Review, 75:*414-424, 1967.

PASAMANICK, BENJAMIN: A comparative study of the behavioral development of Negro infants. *J Genet Psychol, 69:*3-44, 1946.

PASAMANICK, BENJAMIN, AND KNOBLOCH, HILDA: Retrospective studies on the epidemiology of reproductive casualty: old and new. *Merrill-Palmer Quarterly of Behavior and Development, 12*:7-26, 1966.

RHODES, A. J.: Virus infections and congenital malformations. In *Congenital Malformations: Papers and Discussions Presented at the First International Conference on Congenital Malformations.* Philadelphia, Lippincott. 1961, pp. 106-116.

SCHAEFER, E. S.: Does the sampling method produce the negative correlation of mean IQ with age reported by Kennedy, Van De Riet, and White? *Child Dev, 36*:257-259, 1965.

SCHAEFFER, H. R., AND EMERSON, P. E.: Patterns of response to physical contact in early human development. *J Child Psychol Psychiatry, 5*:1-13, 1964a.

SCHAFFER, H. R., AND EMERSON, P. E.: The development of social attachments in infancy. *Monogr Soc Res Child Dev, 29* (3) (*No. 94*), 1964b.

SCRIMSHAW, NEVIN S., AND GORDON, JOHN E.: *Malnutrition, Learning and Behavior.* Cambridge, The M.I.T. Press, 1968.

SIMPSON, WINEA J.: A preliminary report on cigarette smoking and the incidence of prematurity. *Am J Obstet Gyn, 73*:808-815, 1957.

STEWART, R. J. C., AND PLATT, B. S.: Nervous system damage in experimental protein-calorie deficiency. In Scrimshaw and Gordon: *Malnutrition, Learning and Behavior,* Cambridge, The M.I.T. Press, 1968, pp. 168-180.

TIBER, NORMAN, AND KENNEDY, WALLACE A.: The effects of incentives on the intelligence test performance of different social groups. *J Consult Clin Psychol, 28*:187, 1964.

VENKATACHALAM, P. S., AND RAMANATHAN, K. S.: Effect of protein deficiency during gestation and lactation on body weight and composition of offspring. *J Nutr, 84*:38, 1964.

WARKANY, JOSEF: Congenital malformations induced by maternal nutritional deficiency. *J Pediatr, 25*:476-480, 1944.

WARKANY, JOSEF: Etiology of congenital malformations. In *Advances in Pediatrics.* Edited by S. Z. Levine. New York, Interscience. 1947, pp. 1-63.

WHITE, B. L., AND CASTLE, P. W.: Visual exploratory behavior following postnatal handling of human infants. *Percept Mot Skills, 18*:497-502, 1964.

WORTIS, HELEN: Social class and premature birth. *Social Casework, 45*:541-543, 1963.

YARROW, LEON J.: Research in dimensions of early maternal care. *Merrill-Palmer Quarterly, 9*:101-114, 1963.

ZIGLER, EDWARD: Mental retardation: current issues and approaches. In *Review of Child Development Research.* Vol. 2. Edited by Lois W. Hoffman and Martin L. Hoffman. New York, Russell Sage Foundation. 1966, pp. 107-168.

DISCUSSION I

SUSAN W. GRAY, PH.D.

Evidence has been accumulating for many years to suggest the probability that the behavior of all organisms results from the interaction of the developing structure and the environment. We must look at the problem of nature and nurture in this context.

There might be an alternative explanation to the one Dr. Kennedy suggested, though it may be an optimistic hypothesis. As age increased, Dr. Kennedy mentioned the marked drop found in his 1960 testing, a greater drop than is really entirely credible. He pointed out one of the possible factors—that the youngsters were selected on the basis of grade. This, of course, militates against getting a fairly stable intelligence quotient. Possibly one of the reasons he found no IQ loss in his 1965 sample may have been because the school environment is beginning to have some effect, and these youngsters are showing some improvement. One of the interesting things in the intervention project at Peabody (although from the standpoint of research it has created complications) is that just plain, garden-variety school seems to help deprived children. It probably does not provide as much help as the children need, but at least the average, relatively adequate school is beneficial. The control group in our main city, for example, showed a gain of six IQ points during the first year of school. Perhaps one reason Dr. Kennedy did not find a loss in 1965 may have been school is getting a little better.

There are two things to be commented upon rather briefly as adding a little more to our concern with possible environmental factors. First, we might look at immediate situational variables. For four years now we have been working with eighty-seven youngsters who have been tested many times. In terms of this testing, there have been a number of interesting situational variables influencing test performance. One on which we are currently working is the influence of the examiner's race and sex. We picked this up in the work of Irwin Katz (1964). Some know his results with Negro college-age and adolescent boys. Katz finds that the race of the examiner has an influence upon performance; that there is an interaction between the race of the examiner and the amount of stress in the situation. He has recently done work on expectancy set, which also shows an interaction effect. All of these seem to suggest that the performance of the Negro boy (the individual he happened to work with) is vulnerable to changes in race of the examiner and the general situation.

We have been working on something called the Kindergarten Katz at Peabody. The idea is to study race and sex of the examiner in different kinds of test and learning situations. We have combined with Katz's approach some of Harold Stevenson's (1965) rationale on social reinforcement. Judith Phillips (1966), now working at Peabody, has become interested in the race and sex of the experimenter in relationship to the family structure of the deprived child. In working with deprived Negro boys, ages eleven or twelve, she finds that boys from father-absent homes show a different pattern from those from father-present homes. The most potent examiner (or experimenter) for them is the Negro male. You can formulate some hypotheses in terms of identification. The situational aspects of measures of general adequacy are important, particularly with the deprived population, where the individual generally is much less familiar with reacting to a wide range of expectancies and to a wide range of strange adults. Situational factors interact with the type of test, as one might guess. This is true, for example, on the Illinois Test of Psycholinguistic Ability [1], where some subtests are influenced and not others.

Another general comment in circulation pertains to the washout effects in intervention projects with young children. Often, there is considerable amount of unrealistic expectancies in terms of gains in intelligence. These expectancies arise in part out of factors related to test performance. A child who comes from a deprived environment, for example, is not accustomed to strange people or to being put down, as Dr.

---

[1] *The Illinois Test of Psycholinguistic Abilities*, by James J. McCarthy and Samuel A. Kirk, is published by the University of Illinois Institute for Research on Exceptional Children and distributed by the University of Illinois Press.

Kennedy says, with a crayon or pencil and a piece of paper. Naturally, he is not going to do very well on a paper and pencil test. However, place crayons and pencils before him for about ten weeks, with about fifteen adults milling around in the room with him. It would hardly be surprising at the end of the period if the motivational situation in terms of testing is different. So some projects, believing they have changed intelligence, have, instead made more of a change in test adequacy. Another reason why we have comments of washout effects is because one can get a quick change by specific teaching, but as soon as the test content changes (as it will after another year for a young child) the effect may be gone. Intervention projects showing a gain in general adequacy over a long period of time will not fall into this trap. Some intervention projects are producing gains which appear to be relatively lasting. These studies seem to demonstrate that the environment has an influence upon test performance over and beyond the situational factors mentioned. It is important for any investigator interested in changing performance through intervention projects to be highly sensitive to the situational factors which may influence test performance.

REFERENCES

KATZ, I.: Review of evidence to effects of desegregation on the intellectual performance of Negroes. *Amer Psychol, 19*:381-389, 1964.

PHILLIPS, JUDITH: Performance of father-present and father-absent Southern Negro boys on a simple operant task as a function of the race and sex of the experimenter and the type of social reinforcement. Unpublished doctoral dissertation, University of Minnesota, 1966.

STEVENSON, H. W.: Social reinforcement of children's behavior. In Lipsitt, L. P., and Spiker, C. C. (eds.): *Advances in Child Development and Behavior. New York*, Academic Press, 1965, vol. II.

DISCUSSION II

HERBERT W. SMITH, PH.D.

The present speaker completely agrees with all the statements made by Dr. Kennedy. However, parts of a study relevant to the area under consideration will be presented.

Some data strongly suggest some of our measurements in regard to minority group children are a long way from being understood. Dr. Ted May and this speaker have been very interested in studying the influence of the examiner on the Stanford-Binet (Form L-M) scores of "culturally deprived" children. Both have collected some data, and have borrowed quite a bit from investigators who were willing to share their information. Both have been basically working with two samples, the first sample including 435 Stanford-Binet scores of four-year-old Negro children. Six examiners were involved in this sample. The second sample included 316 six-year-old Negro children tested by eight examiners. All the children who served as subjects in these two samples lived in Memphis, Tennessee.

The two investigators have been analyzing the data of these two samples for examiner variability. By looking at the first sample, preliminary ideas regarding examiner variability were obtained. The second sample was collected to follow up some of the ideas suggested by the first analysis.

These two samples were connected by retesting sixty-four children at age six who had been tested at age four. The test-retest correlation was .48. This correlation is lower than one would expect; some authors have reported correlation in the high 70's for the same time period, test and population.

It was felt the low correlation was more of a result of examiner bias than changes in performance of the population during the time between testings.

To study this question, eight examiners with varying qualifications were selected to administer the Stanford-Binet (Form L-M) to minority group children. Table I shows the background information on the examiners used in this study. They varied in sex, race and familiarity with the test administered. Two examiners had previous testing experience; the remaining testers were either certified guidance counselors or graduate students in psychology. In this study, the primary interest was in the relationship between testing experience and scores elicited from Negro children.

Table II reports the results of breaking the data into two parts: the first and second half of testing, for each examiner,

TABLE I
BACKGROUND INFORMATION ON EXAMINERS

Examiner Number	Age	Sex	Race	Testing Experience	Degrees	Occupation
1	44	F	Cau.	2 testing courses	BS, MS	Kindergarten teacher (4 yrs.)
2	24	M	Cau.	6 months	BA	Graduate student (Psychology)
3	25	M	Cau.	2 testing courses	BA, MA	Instructor in Psychology
4	24	F	Cau.	None	BA	Graduate student (Psychology)
5	47	M	Negro	None	BA, MS	Guidance counselor
6	41	F	Negro	None	BA, MA	Guidance counselor
7	23	M	Cau.	None	BA	Graduate student (Psychology)
8	22	F	Cau.	None	BA	Graduate student (Psychology)

TABLE II
MEANS AND VARIANCES—STANFORD-BINET (L-M)
FIRST HALF AND SECOND HALF OF TESTING

Examiner Number	Sex	N_1	N_2	M_1	M_2	S_1	S_2
1	F	21	21	86.9	81.1	159.5	104.7
4	F	22	21	85.5	81.4	170.4	53.1
6	F	21	20	93.1	88.2	143.9	160.3
8	F	12	13	84.2	81.4	146.3	81.4
2	M	28	28	83.4	86.6	129.6	119.9
3	M	25	25	84.4	88.2	127.8	66.2
5	M	21	22	87.8	86.1	64.2	46.8
7	M	8	8	82.4	88.6	219.1	138.5
Overall Means				86.2	85.2	137.6	93.0

regardless of the total number of children tested. By dividing the data in this manner, it was hoped to identify the influence of the experience of the examiner.

The most striking result in this table is that by arbitrarily breaking this data in half, one can see a significant reduction in the pooled variance estimated. Even the more experienced examiner elicited scores which appear to be estimating two population variance parameters during the two testing periods. The pooled variance estimate was 137.6 during the first half of testing. During the second half of testing, the pooled variance estimate was 93.0. This shift is visible in seven of the eight examiners used in this study.

Another interesting factor in the data was the shift in mean scores elicited during the two testing periods. Female examiners elicited significantly lower scores during the second half of testing. Male examiners elicited numerically larger scores during the second half of testing. The consistency of these shifts in sample statistics computed cannot be attributed to sampling error.

Something must be said about the initial samples studied. In the sample of 435 four-year-old Negro children tested by six experienced examiners, the shift in variance estimate is present. The data was broken into the first, second, and finally third of "section" testing and tested the assumption of equal variance between examiners. The Bartlett's test was significant beyond the .01 level for the first third of testing and nonsignificant for the other two-thirds.

In summary, the data with regard to the variance estimates produced by six experienced and eight inexperienced examiners administering the Stanford-Binet (Form L-M) to four and six year-old Negro children indicate both samples have significant fluctuation in pooled variance estimates between the early and late phase of testing.

Some additional sources of examiner variability visible in the samples are also present. The sex of the examiner was significant in the four-year sample, and marginally significant in the six-year sample. The significance of race of the examiner has already been discussed by Dr. Gray. There was a significant interaction between the sex of the examiner and the sex of the subject in early phases of testing. However, this factor seems to fall out as the examiner becomes more experienced.

In addition to the overall shifts in the data discussed previously, some of the examiners elicited scores which formed certain consistent patterns. Related to the testing "style" of the examiner these patterns are over and above such considerations as race, sex and experience of the examiner. Any attempt at specifying testing "style" at this time is premature, but some ideas in this area must be discussed. Specifically, three testing "styles" helping to account for some of the examiner differences in the samples studied, will be discussed here.

The first style may be called "on the job." This seems to be characteristic of an examiner who is responding to the pressure of turning out a lot of test scores. This examiner, after a period of time, can administer the Stanford-Binet (Form L-M) in a ten to fifteen minute period. An examiner who falls into this classification elicited scores significantly lower than the other examiners. This "style" was characteristic of some graduate students and other examiners in the samples studied.

The second style, which may be called "old reliable," is usually characteristic of an examiner who, after a period of time, comes to expect a certain score. The scores elicited by this examiner show a striking similarity to repeated measures of the same subject. The mean and variance estimates of this type of examiner are very close to the other examiners, except very little variance is visible between successive samples tested.

The last testing style is the "social critic." Several examiners elicited mean and variance estimates which seem to be a protest against social conditions. Mean estimates of these examiners are seven to ten points above or below what would be expected when the sex, race and experience of the examiner have been controlled.

A great deal of what has been said today is speculative in nature. Some areas of examiner variability needing exploration have been suggested. However, enough evidence is present to indicate a great deal of the problems psychologists have encountered in using the Stanford-Binet in predicting future performance, or in diagnostic work, is related to examiner variability.

Can you imagine what the results of a test-retest study would be if the first tests were administered by a Caucasian male graduate student who subscribed to the "on the job" style of testing, after which the subjects were retested by a Negro female examiner "social critic"? The mean difference would be at least ten points. The race, sex and testing "style" of the examiner would combine to produce low scores on the first test, and high scores on the retest. If this suggested study had been used to evaluate a program designed to improve performance, then a significant result would have been obtained.

In addition to the variations between examiners, the shift in variance and means for an examiner with testing experience could also produce confounded results. The results of the sample studies would indicate that as an examiner gains in testing experience, his variance estimates are substantially reduced. This reduction in variance estimate would contribute to a small error term computed during the post-testing period. This effect could produce a significant result, especially when one of the major variables would be the experience of the examiner.

The possibility of studying examiner variability has only recently been feasible because of the large research programs currently under way. They afford the opportunity to study scores elicited by examiners on the same population over a long period of time. Most of the children who were subjects in these studies are minority group children. Therefore, many people feel this population of children are the only ones influenced to any great degree by examiner bias. However, when we reanalyze some of the scores elicited from other groups, we will find the same general picture.

VI

INTELLECTUAL EVALUATION OF CHILDREN WITH MAJOR SENSORY DEFICIT

JERRY N. BOONE, PH.D.

THIS PAPER will deal with problems which the clinical psychologist encounters when he is called upon to assess the intellectual ability of children who are deaf or blind. Many of us have found our way through graduate training and several years of experience with children in clinical settings without encountering many who are deaf or blind. Many of us, when called upon to serve these children, are reluctant to do so. We are discouraged by the obvious difficulty of communicating with them and in utilizing the familiar tests in which we have confidence. We know there are specialized tests which some people use, plus alterations which frequently are made in the use of the more common instruments. Unfortunately, a considerable amount of the literature which deals with tests and testing of the blind and deaf, is not found in the usual psychological publications, but in such journals as the *Journal of Speech and Hearing Disorders; American Annals of the Deaf; Volta Review; Outlook for the Blind* and the *Journal of Rehabilitation*.

Just how skillful are we at making judgments about the abilities of these children? A student in the California State School for the Deaf remained in a hospital for the retarded for five years because of a Stanford-Binet IQ of 29, before being "paroled" on the basis of a performance IQ of 113, many years later (Vernon and Brown, 1964). In a research project in another state school for the deaf, childern were evaluated with five different performance tests. The IQ's varied widely from test to test, in one instance as much as 53 points in this population of apparently well-adjusted children (Birch and Birch, 1951).

To be considered in this paper are some alternatives which the psychologist has in choosing tests for the deaf and the blind, some problems he may encounter in interacting with the child during testing, and some methodological issues involved in perfecting tests for children with sensory handicaps.

Newland (1963) has an excellent review of the issues involved in testing the sensory handicapped. He feels we are so limited in intellectual measurement of the deaf and the blind that we should lean a great deal further toward dependence on physical correlates of mental growth, such as bone growth and cephalic indices. We certainly would like to believe that our tests, while measuring only present functioning, allow us to make some reasonable inferences about a child's intellectual potential. The sensory and experiential deprivation imposed upon a deaf or a blind child no doubt detract markedly from the actualizing of his intellectual potential. Myklebust (1960) states this very nicely when he calls mental development the ". . . reciprocal of limitation in language acquisition." This kind of reasoning, of course, allows for the most charitable interpretation of the low scores commonly found among groups of deaf and blind children when tested on instruments devised for a normal population. Myklebust believes that deafness compromises measured intelligence to the extent that it is never possible to compare deaf and hearing populations with respect to global intelligence. He points out that verbal tests have no place even with those persons whose deafness occurred since language was acquired. The assumption that they can comprehend through speech-reading and through-reading, that they can express themselves orally and in writing, does not always hold.

If children with sensory handicaps must be evaluated so differently from the normal, the question arises as to what criteria are to be used in validating tests constructed specifically for them, or in determining the validity of the common tests when used with the deaf or the blind. One point of view (Graham and Shapiro, 1953) is that since deaf must live in a hearing world and compete with the hearing, they should be mesaured by the same instruments with only the most necessary modifications, and be judged by the norms applying to the hearing. An opposing point of view, stated by Newland (1963) points up the uniqueness of the school and training experiences of those who have sensory handicaps as well as the fact that our tests are presumed to predict their performances in those unique situations. Educational measures to which the deaf and blind are exposed are so different from the normal that we would not expect the usual intelligence tests interpreted by the usual norms to do a very good job of predicting. If we are to use tests specifically devised for the deaf and blind, or if we are to restandardize those parts of the usual instruments which can be used, we must identify criteria of learning ability within that special school situation against which to validate the tests.

The criterion problem with the deaf and the blind is much more confused than with the normal. Let us illustrate the problem with the deaf. Just what is academic success for the deaf? Does it consist of academic success in an oral program where no manual communication is allowed? Does it consist of success in acquiring oral language and understanding of oral language? Or does it consist of success in acquiring the vocational skills for which even the bright deaf person may be better suited than he is for an academic career? The point is, with so many different kinds of educational programs for the sensory handicapped, it should not be surprising that we will have difficulty in constructing tests which measure learning ability and predict academic achievement in a variety of settings. On the other hand, if we agree that the deaf and blind must be measured in relation to their normal peers, we must predict their success with far less than we would like to have in the way of test results, nonverbal results only in the case of the deaf and oral verbal results in the case of the blind.

In the practical situation, when called upon to test the deaf and blind, we simply must decide whether we will use whatever parts possible of the commonly used tests and make estimates from these, or use tests with which we have little experience and have, perhaps, reason to doubt.

Using parts of tests in this situation (just as in the situation where we do so to conserve time) has its drawbacks. Obviously, when we adapt a test by omitting parts and then correct or prorate, it is assumed each item in the test has equivalent measurement value, an assumption hard to defend. Furthermore, there is a question of whether the part given a particular child is likely to be related to the thing we want to predict. For example, we may be restricted to the use of performance items only in evaluating the deaf; yet it is the verbal portions of tests, such as the Wechsler, which correlate best with school achievement in a normal population. We may feel considerably more comfortable in the case of the blind to whom we can administer verbal parts of the test, such as the Wechsler. But here relationships between verbal IQ's and school achievement have been, for the most part, derived from normally seeing populations. If educational criteria for the blind are not the same, and if the educational process for the blnid includes a great deal less of the academic subjects and more vocational training, it's necessary to know how the verbal Wechsler score correlates with the achievement of *blind* children in a school program *for* the blind.

Evidence of validity of test parts with the blind is somewhat scarce. Work done on the Wechsler Verbal Scale with relatively small numbers of children in residential schools for the blind (Scholl, 1953) yielded results supportive in a construct validity sense in that scores among this group ranged from 82 to 115, with a median of 94. Further support for this use of the Wechsler lay in the fact that the same population of children had a median IQ of 95 on the Hayes-Binet.

The Hayes test is, in itself, a use of the "part" approach. Efforts have been made to modify the Binet scale for use with the blind since 1914 (Erwin, 1914, Haines, 1916). Hayes' particular selection of Binet items was collected in 1930 (Hayes, 1930). It was revised during the next ten years and administered to some twenty-three hundred pupils from residential schools for the blind (Hayes, 1941, 1950). Test results from these school-age children were encouraging in that the test discriminated among blind children, yielding a distribution quite similar to the usual distribution of intelligence. There was a mean IQ of 99, with a standard deviation ranging from 15 to 23, Yet, Hayes pointed out a number of shortcomings of the test as a means of estimating intelligence of the blind at all ages, in all ranges of ability. Because the test was standardized on a residential school population, there were very few children below school age. Also, the Binet Test from which it was taken provides a much smaller pool of verbal items from which to select at pre-school ages than at higher age levels. Another objection voiced by Hayes was that the test contained too few verbal items at the adolescent level to give a good measurement of bright older children.

Some objections to a test such as the Hayes, which utilizes only verbal items, center around the belief that the blind as a group suffer in the ability to conceptualize. There is good research evidence to bear out that belief. For example, Rubin (1964) found blind adults doing more poorly on such abstract tasks as proverbs than seeing adults with equal Hayes IQ scores were doing. Newland (1963) stated that the blind's difficulty with abstract concepts is probably due to limited experience rather than a special conceptual disability. He insisted many of the verbal items from the Binet and Wechsler demand concepts (e.g., color) which the blind are handicapped in learning. He pointed out that tactual and kinesthetic abilities are very important in the blind child's learning, and that a test used to predict success should measure these abilities. He has begun construction of a nonverbal test for blind children. There is other mention in the literature of ingenious means of devising such things as Kohs-type blocks with smooth and rough surfaces, for use with a blind population (Wattron, 1956).

The existence of many different performance tests of intelligence has meant that psychologists have not resorted to using parts of tests with the deaf as often as with the blind. Yet some subtests on the Wechsler Performance Scale have lent themselves so easily to presentation through pantomime that psychologists accustomed to that instrument have found it quite useful with the deaf. Graham and Shapiro (1953) for example, found a group of deaf children to achieve a Wechsler Performance IQ only five points lower than a group of hearing children who had Goodenough scores equal to that of the deaf group. Since the hearing children had responded to regular oral instructions and the deaf to pantomime, these investigators concluded the Wechsler Performance Scale can easily be adapted to use with deaf children.

All the well known performance tests, as well as some lesser known ones, have been used with deaf children, and a broad review of the uses of these with the deaf has been published by Vernon and Brown (1964). Evidently, the two most commonly used are the Arthur Adaptation of the Leiter International Performance Scale and the Nebraska Test of Learning Aptitudes for Young Deaf Children (commonly called the Hiskey Test). As the name implies, the Hiskey Test was constructed and standardized for the deaf. The Leiter Scale, on the other hand, was intended as a culture-free test of intelligence for use with hearing persons. However, the fact that it was standardized without verbal instructions led easily to its use with the deaf.

One who is accustomed to the Stanford-Binet would find the Hiskey Test almost familiar. It consists of a rather bulky 124 parts with eleven types of tests, including such familiar tasks as paper-folding and block-stacking. It was standardized on about 500 children (Sloan, 1959) between the ages of four and ten, on the basis of percentage passing at age levels. As is frequently the case, the principal claim to validity is a correlation of .83 with Binet scores on hearing children. A point of interest in interpreting Hiskey "learning quotients" (as the IQ-type score is referred to) is in Hiskey's statement that the average quotient for deaf children would be in the mid-90's, if one used the norms collected on hearing children (Hiskey, 1956). Even though Hiskey's effort to standardize a test on a sample of the deaf population is highly commendable, it must be remembered his standardization sample (including only children in schools for the deaf) was possibly deficient at the lower end of the intellectual distribution, and that norms are available on this test only for children between the ages of four and ten.

One of the appeals of the Leiter scale for use with the deaf is that it is standardized without verbal instructions. A further attractive feature is that its norms extend down as low as two years, it is relatively easily administered and fairly quickly comprehended by the deaf child. Each item over the entire range of the instrument is administered by presentation of a wooden frame into which the subject places blocks in an order dictated by a strip placed in the frame for that particular item. Like the Hiskey, it is an age scale. Evidence for the validity of the Leiter scale in its 1929 edition, its 1940 revision, and its 1948 modification by Arthur is primarily in terms of correlation with the Stanford-Binet (Leiter, ...). Despite reasonably good correlation with the Stanford-Binet, the Leiter appears to have given consistently lower average scores than the Binet when used with a hearing population (Beverly and Bensberg, 1952; Orgel and Dreger, 1955). In fact, the manual itself states, without further explanation, that the mean IQ score is 95. Birch and Birch have conducted studies (1951, 1956) which get at the issue of the Leiter's validity in assessing the ability of deaf children. Children in a school for the deaf were given the Leiter Scale, the Wechsler Performance Scale, the Arthur Point Scale, the Hiskey Test, the Goodenough; scores were compared. There was a distinct pattern revealed in which the Leiter score was consistently the lowest of the five tests, while the Hiskey was among the highest. In their second study (1956) the Birches compared both Leiter IQ's and supervising teachers' ratings of the intelligence of institutionized deaf children, with the later achievement of those children. The Leiter score correlated with achievement rating at .71, while the teachers' estimates of ability correlated with achievement at .82. It appears, then, the scale has some usefulness in predicting school achievement, at least in the particular deaf-school program used in the studies. Also, when used with the deaf, the scale yields consistently lower scores than most other performance tests.

The scant evidence on this subject suggests the Wechsler Performance Scale may be as useful as either of the commonly used whole-performance tests in measuring the intellectual ability of deaf children in the age range where it can be used. The Hiskey Test represents one of the rare instances in which a test is constructed and standardized for a deaf population; with further standardization, it may prove to be extremely useful in some kinds of institutional settings for the deaf. The advantage of the Leiter scale lies in its face validity, its ease of administration and the fact that norms go down as low as two years. Both the Hiskey Test and the Leiter Test appear to yield mean IQ scores in the 90's, which should be regarded carefully in making test interpretations. Intelligence scores from these tests should not be utilized without operational reference to this eccentricity of the two instruments in comparison with the usual intelligence test. It should be noted that with IQ means in the mid-90's and standard deviations near 20, scores on these tests in the IQ range of 75 to 95 represent, presumably, the same population as that represented in the range 85 to 100 on the typical intelligence test.

Let us look for a moment at the question of whether inference concerning abnormal central nervous system-functioning can legitimately be made from intelligence tests with the deaf and blind. Can CNS abnormality be inferred from the deaf or blind child's showing comparative deficiency in certain areas of functioning? Or is there something about deafness and blindness themselves which cause subjects to do poorly on tasks often associated with organic involvement in the hearing and seeing population, such as memory, abstracting ability and visual-motor coordination? Newland (1963) asserts there is no research relative to the validity of psychological tests used in identifying brain damage in the deaf and blind. In work previously mentioned by Rubin (1960) there was some indication the blind do more poorly on such abstract tasks as proverbs, than do the seeing. Myklebust (1960) reviews studies of the relationship between deafness and the abstraction process, as well as studies of the relationhip between deafness and memory. He concludes (although evidence is conflicting) that inferiority in some measures of abstraction is a condition secondary to the language limitation of the deaf, who characteristically do more poorly in some tests of memory than the hearing. If memory and abstraction suffer in these populations by virtue of the sensory handicap alone, then deficiency showing up in these areas of intelligence tests may not indicate a CNS abnormality beyond the sensory. It may well be, however, that errors on drawing tasks and reproductions of designs commonly associated with organic problems are valid with the deaf. A study by Furth (1963) investigating the visual gestalt function and reproducing designs, found these not to be affected by deafness.

In addition to the problems of selecting tests for the sensory handicapped, what difficulties is the psychologist likely to encounter in the administration of a test and the behavior of a child? In communicating with the deaf child, one needs to be quite aware of the degree of hearing loss. A child with a hearing loss as great as 45 to 65 d.b. may appear to hear adequately. He may be picking up enough of what he hears and of the situation itself, to respond at a superficial level as if he understands. However, a child with this degree of hearing loss has lost what Myklebust (1960) calls the "scanning" function. He tends to give all sound equal attention; thus, his comprehension may be spotty and render invalid any tests given even partly with verbal instructions. This is of particular importance in dealing with the Wechsler Performance Scale in which the administration through pantomime "extends" the examiner quite a bit. The deaf child often appears to be accustomed to trying to look bright and responsive when he is spoken to, accustomed to smiling and nodding, which can fake the examiner into thinking that a test given with loud verbal instruction is getting through to the child. Obtaining the child's trust, reassuring him about leaving his mother, and rewarding him enough to keep him motivated during a long testing session are particularly difficult for the psychologist who cannot easily become animated. Many examiners seem to be more able to relate to the deaf child if they talk with him as they normally would, while depending entirely on gesture and touch to communicate with him; perhaps the child responds to that which is natural for the examiner. Some persons, accustomed to testing deaf children (Vernon and Brown, 1964) doubt the validity of any timed items with the deaf who appear to some to have difficulty in forming time concepts.

The blind child presents no communicating problem of such proportions as those with the deaf child. However, some of the behavioral characteristics of the blind, the gesturing and posturing called "blindisms," may be quite disruptive of the testing process. Problems imposed by these behaviors are well described by Bauman (1952).

In evaluation of the deaf and blind, the psychologist has specialized intelligence tests and parts of familiar ones at his disposal. He recognizes these tests leave a good deal to be desired. Some have been standardized on a population of normal children. Even though they predict reasonably good success for the normal reasonably well, we wonder whether the tests predict a child's learning in a school program which is quite different. Other tests have norms drawn from deaf and blind samples more restricted than preferable with respect to number, age range, and ability range. The tests available often do not tap important abilities such as the language potential of the child who is likely to go into a school where oral language is the principal goal; or the tactual and kinesthetic abilities of the blind child who is likely to be taught nonacademic vocational skills.

The problem demands identifying the kinds of ability significant for the achievement of the deaf and blind, and demands these abilities be the ones measured. These may or may not be the abilities which make up the presently usable instruments. This cannot be done until we first identify reasonable success criteria for the blind and deaf from among the goals of diverse special educational programs. Until these tasks are accomplished, the psychologist cannot place the usual amount of confidence in his intelligence test results, and must insist that other correlates of mental growth be given heavier-than-usual weight in prediction.

REFERENCES

1. BAUMAN, M. K.: Diagnostic procedures in rehabilitation of the blind. *J Rehab*, 7-11, 1952.
2. BEVERLY, L., AND BENSBERG, G. J.: A comparison of the Leiter, the Cornell-Coxe, and the Stanford-Binet with mental defectives. *Amer J Ment Defic*, 57:89-91, 1952.
3. BIRCH, J. R., AND BIRCH, J. W.: The Leiter International Performance

Scale as an aid in the psychological study of the deaf. *Amer Ann Deaf*, 96:502-511, 1951.

4. BIRCH, J. R., AND BIRCH, J. W.: Predicting school achievement in young deaf children. *Amer Ann Deaf*, 101:348-352, 1956.

5. FURTH, H. G., AND MENDEZ, R. A.: The influence of language and age on Gestalt laws of perception. *Amer J Psychol*, 76:74-81, 1963.

6. GRAHAM, E. E., AND SHAPIRO, E.: Use of the performance scale of the Wechsler Intelligence Scale for Children with the deaf child. *J Consult Psychol*, 17:396-398, 1953.

7. HAINES, T. H.: A psychological survey of the Ohio State School for the Blind. *Outlook for the Blind*, 9:88-92, 1916.

8. HAYES, S. P.: Terman's condensed guide for the Stanford revision of the Binet-Simon intelligence tests adapted for use with the blind. *Perkins Institute Publications, No. 4*, 1930.

9. HAYES, S. P.: *Contributions to a Psychology of Blindness*. New York, American Foundation for the Blind, 1941.

10. HAYES, S. P.: Measuring the intelligence of the blind. In Zahl, P. A. (Ed.): *Blindness*. Princeton, Princeton U., 1950.

11. HISKEY, M. K., A study of the intelligence of deaf and hearing children. *Amer Ann Deaf*, 101:329-339, 1956.

12. IRWIN, R. B.: A Binet scale for the blind. *Outlook for the Blind*, 8:95-97, 1914.

13. LEITER, G. R.: *Part I of the Manual for the 1948 Revision of the Leiter International Performance Scale*. Beverly Hills, Calif., Western Psychological Services, (no publication date).

14. MYKLEBUST, H. R.: *The Psychology of Deafness*. New York, Grune and Stratton, 1960.

15. NEWLAND, T. E.: Psychological assessment of exceptional children and youth. In Cruickshank, W. M. (ed.): *Psychology of Exceptional Children and Youth*. Englewood Cliffs, N. J., Prentice-Hall, 1963.

16. ORGEL, A. R., AND DREGER, R. M.: A comparative study of the Arthur-Leiter and the Stanford-Binet Intelligence Scales. *J Genet Psychol*, 86:359-365, 1955.

17. RUBIN, E. J.: *Abstract Functioning of the Blind*. American Foundation for the blind. American Foundation for the Blind Research Series, No. 11, 1964.

18. SCHOLL, G.: Intelligence tests for visually handicapped children. *Exceptional Child*, 20:116-123, 1953.

19. SLOAN, W.: Nebraska Test of Learning Aptitudes. In Buros, O. K. (ed.): *Fifth Mental Measurements Yearbook*, New York, Gryphon, 1959.

20. VERNON, M., AND BROWN, D. W.: A guide to psychological tests and testing procedures in the evaluation of deaf and hard-of-hearing children. *J Speech Hearing Dis*, 29:414-423, 1964.

21. WATTRON, J. B.: A suggested performance test of intelligence. *The New Outlook for the Blind,* 50:115-121, 1956.

DISCUSSION I

MARTIN A. MENDELSON, PH.D.

Dr. Boone's paper has raised some provocative questions. The field of working with handicapped children, specifically children showing sensory lack or deprivation in the area of hearing and blindness, is indeed an important one.

There is a problem here in terms of what our goals are. Our interest in predicting how this handicapped child, blind or deaf, will function in society among people who are not so handicapped could be important. Therefore, it is almost compelling to use the available psychological measures, taking into account the limited range of performance the sensory handicap itself may exert upon the child's performance. Implicitly, in doing so, we are trying to determine whether this individual can become a functioning member of society. Nevertheless, in a sense, he is isolated by our deliberately excluding certain types of occupations in which the sensory modality he lacks are required. The development of specific job families for the handicapped is represented in the work of the Office of Vocational Rehabilitation and the U.S. Office of Education. These efforts, naturally and unavoidably, tend to promote further isolation of the handicapped in the world at large. The word "isolation" must be put in quotes. The very nature of these children's handicaps causes them to be isolated to a certain extent. For example, the richness of appreciation for music or for art in particular is something a child auricularly handicapped at birth will never experience. All of the modalities we possess intact combine in giving us percepts and concepts of the world at large. It is impossible to convey, to a deaf child (one who has been deaf since birth) the essence of music, and it is impossible to convey to a blind child the essence and appreciation of art.

When we have to test across other intact modalities for these handicapped children, another question arises, in terms of the relationship of these modalities to intelligence. How far can we go? Is not the range of tasks being offered somewhat limited? And are they also somewhat irrelevant, depending on our goals? Considering the degree of his handicap, can we merge the handicapped child into society, or must we virtually isolate him in some kind of useful occupation which will tend to improve or ameliorate the condition to a certain extent? Our psychological instruments are not that precise. There are errors in sampling; in a psychological test, we are taking only a sampling of behavior at that time, used in various ways to assess the intellectual status of the child and dependent upon the nature of the tests used. The element of prediction has been much overstressed. Most tests can be used as diagnostic and predictive, but when we get into the blind and deaf, the criteria for prediction must be reiterated. As Dr. Boone has indicated, the specific kind of criteria in terms of their social implications, their work implications, and their educational implications have to be clearly specified.

The quality of individual differences among the visually handicapped and the auricularly handicapped child has to be taken into account. There is a case in Maryland of a child who has retrolental fibroplasia. The boy has done remarkably well, despite his blindness. This child rides a bicycle. He is at the top of his class, and has been skipped several grades because he is able to cope with the various kinds of things we consider important in the assessment of intelligence in the normal child. If he were to be tested with the usual examinations reserved for the blind, trouble would arise in making a valid assessment, especially if he were restricted to the specific tests for the visually handicapped now available. Another case is of a blind lawyer who does quite well. The degree of his handicap (i.e. acquired, or born with it) has something to do with his adjustment to society. It is imaginable that the intact child who, later on, is deprived of one of his modalities by some kind of accident or disease, has a headstart on those children who are born with these defects. In another way, this child is at a disadvantage because he must cope, again, with the process of retraining and relearning the use of other modalities.

When it comes to intelligence, if we are modality-oriented and want to use substitute examinations correlating highly with intelligence but involving emphasis on other intact modalities, we would be very limited. It is impossible to envisage in a blind child, for example, a test of kinesthetic sensitivity or tactile sensitivity which can be broadened to carry it up to highly abstract levels. We develop our "gimmicks" to a great extent, which sometimes tends to make them highly artificial; the more gimmicks we develop, the less valid the test sometimes seems to be. The reliance upon correlations perhaps is slightly extreme in our profession without the additional qualifications of some kind of assessment criteria which, as Newland (1963) points out, are sorely needed.

As psychologists, we are familiar with the layman's concept of the IQ and the tendency in many instances to allot more weight to it than it deserves. There must also be additional criteria of an evaluative, a qualitative kind of judgment of the child's performance in connection with a test, and in connection with many other types of information. In personal experience with the Collaborative Project,[1] our interest is in the normal child only insofar as deviations from the norm can be detected. But we are also forced to follow this procedure because the clinical, the intuitive, qualitative evaluations obviously do not lend themselves to any kind of objective structure and standardization. To a great extent, valid observations of deviations from the norm are dependent upon the experience of the individual clinician, the psychologist, the psychiatrist, or neurologist. Such observations are also dependent upon his own particular conscious or, perhaps, unconscious bias, and finally, on the type of children and their variations in the types of children he sees in clinical practice.

Among the most important things to be defined are the goals and objectives of our psychological tests and assessments in connection with their application to the handicapped child. If we are interested in turning this individual into a functioning member in society at large, we are almost compelled to use

---

[1]Collaborative Project on Cerebral Palsy, Mental Retardation and other Neurological and Sensory Disorders of Infancy and Childhood sponsored by the National Institute of Neurological Diseases and Blindness, National Institutes of Health.

the kinds of tests for which we establish norms with normal children. If we want to make these individuals function within the limitations of their sensory deprivation, then another testing approach (which obviously leads to a form of isolation) must be used.

REFERENCES

NEWLAND, T. E.: Psychological assessment of exceptional children and youth. In Cruickshank, W. M. (ed.): *Psychology of Exceptional Children and Youth.* Englewood Cliffs, N. J., Prentice-Hall, 1963.

VII

THE ROLE OF INTERPRETIVE PARENT INTERVIEW IN DIAGNOSES OF CHILDREN

WENTWORTH QUAST, PH.D.

Today I'm not going to wear the hat of a Minnesota dust bowl empiricist; I'm going to play clinician. Work in general in mental retardation is most likely involved with attending to immediate problems presented by the child. But in an institute such as this, we might take a broader look than is possible in our everyday stamping out of brush fires. If we are the experts in human relations we have set ourselves up to be, then we are amiss if, in the course of diagnosis and treatment of a handicapped child, we fail to meet the unmet needs of the troubled parent. Consideration of parental feelings, knowledge of the problem, and the parents' expectations are as important as a detailed study of the child—literally a 50-50 proposition. The counseling of parents in very adequate fashion is part and parcel of the operation of many agencies, especially day-care centers. However, it is overlooked often enough for parents to be unwittingly consigned to years of frustration and half-doubts.

In 1958 there was a Woods School conference held in Minneapolis, ostensibly for the purpose of talking about the counseling of parents. But, now, ten years later, though there has been some discussion on this, in my judgment not a great deal has been done about the problem. As Leo Kanner (Johns Hopkins) says: "Delinquency—everybody talks about it [and he seems to be tired of this] but not enough people do something about it."

Reynolds (1953) has reported two studies in which parents of severely retarded children (under IQ 50) were interviewed in the home and by questionnaire. One group had children in public school special classes for the severely retarded, and another group consisted of children not in public school classes. Parents were asked such questions as:

> What gave you the first reason to think that your child might be a little slower in developing than other children?
> What made you sure?
> Where did you first turn for help? (And here, interestingly it was as often the teacher as the M.D.)
> Whom else have you seen about your child?
> What person or agency has been most valuable to you in understanding your child?

In general, both studies were summarized as follows:

> It is shown that parents have often not succeeded in obtaining early diagnosis of their children's condition, and that usually they have not had early help in planning for the care and training of the children. Most parents prefer keeping these children at home even into the adult years (and incidentally, I know of no long-term follow-up into adulthood) but they look to the school program for help in developing *social skills* and self-help. The total information presented gives strong testimony to the need for professional workers to improve their skills in dealing with these parents.

It should be noted that in these studies directly concerned with parents any mention of counseling with parents is for the most part limited to questions having to do with the child, the retardation *per se,* but not with parents' feelings and family integration.

According to Dr. Harriet Blodgett (1959), Director of the Sheltering Arms (a research day care center in Minneapolis), "The critical life event of having a retarded child is a *continuing* critical life event—not one that happens and then is over and ended." Who is to carry the burden for this continuing care, and the responsibility to parents in particular, is by no means clear. Currently, the President's Panel has suggested that a prime problem is the necessity of delegating the responsibility of continuing contact to one social agency. It seems the public schools do not seem to be able to afford such staffing; administratively they are likely to see it as other than a proper educational function. Medicine and public health nursing, for example, are unlikely to provide this kind of care; so it would seem county welfare boards and social workers are the most likely source of help. The difficulty here, as is the case in so many disciplines, is to be a degree person who ends up as a supervisor, with the result that there are no worker bees. There is a hopeful trend in some areas. For example, recently the Armed Forces have trained technicians in a wide variety of responsibilities, even down to the field of surgery and into psychometry. It may well result in similar experiments to train housewives as psychotherapists to help solve this casework problem.

There is much overlapping of functions among the number of disciplines working with children, plus the decentralization of facilities. It may eventuate that a local, city Children's Bureau may be the solution, acting as a clearing house for centralizing the total management of problems. In any event, currently, many of us from different disciplines and settings deal every day with families with a retarded or a brain-syndrome child. Since it is likely no one discipline will be assigned the responsibility for these problems, we should do our best in the training of all personnel likely to be involved. Not too many years ago in our own hospital training center, we very zealously guarded our training and protected the name of clinical psychologist. In recent years it has been my effort to train school psychologists, teachers, and to open our doors—these people are going to do this anyway, so the more we can help any discipline involved, the better.

In the area of research efforts, it seems unfortunate that with all the monies being spent in the areas of retardation and neurology, that so very little is being spent in this whole area of parental and family needs. The remarks which follow will be aimed at this need, as well as at some of the typical twists parental involvement may take in an effort to help us enlarge the scope of our attack on retardation and cerebral dysfunction.

Since semantics—how we say what we say to parents—can be just as important as any detailed medical study, we might clarify right in the beginning even the very title of this Institute. For example, in talking about brain damage, we run into trouble when discussing this with parents, and sometimes, even in our communication with colleagues. Most of my child neurologist associates always ask a psychologist, "What do you mean when you talk about damage?" A preferable term is cerebral dysfunction. There are probably twelve to fifteen terms; it's high time we select one without the irrevocable connotation that "damage" has.

Also, the phrase "with particular emphasis on associated brain damage" will connote to some the idea of brain damage as an additional or accompanying condition. I don't wish to get into the old organic-functional-dichotomy problem, but with the modern medical methods of saving children, base-rate-wise it is possible that cerebral dysfunction is the most likely and parsimonious etiology for retardation, irrespective of degree.

There is little time at this stage, at least, to discuss theoretical formulations of retardation; obviously some were expressed, but I'd like to refer you to one. Excluding detail, this is a reference from Dr. Leo Kanner (a favorite teacher of mine) in which he describes three conditions of mental retardation: *"absolute,"* *"relative,"* and *"apparent."* If you are interested in all three, you can check Kanner's book. My interest is in the middle area— relative retardation. Just to quote this one, *"Relative"* consists of individuals whose limitations are definitely related to the standards of the particular society which surrounds them. In less complex, less intellectually centered societies, they would have no trouble in attaining and retaining equality of realizable ambition.

"The particular society" can be limited even to small societies—the family or neighborhood, for example. One of the common problems is of a child who is relatively retarded in a bright family; or a child who goes to a suburban school where the mean IQ is 116 in the whole district, but this fellow has an IQ of 90, so he is *relatively* retarded. Recently, I had a superintendent who said of a child with an 89 IQ that he had no place in the school for this child (if you can imagine). But this was literally true—everybody was advanced-program, college-oriented, and the child actually could not be educated in this particular system.

I am also very interested in some of the visiting firemen

who have come through our institution from England, who impressed me with their attitude in general toward IQ. It is a relative matter to them, like height and weight, and they don't give the absolute value we place on it.

To return to the parents: There is some objective research, although not a great deal, on the effects of a retarded or handicapped child on family integration. I would recommend the two monographs by Bernard Farber (1959) for example. A recent study by Dr. Cooper showed significantly higher divorce rates, emotionally disturbed sibs and other evidence of disturbance in the families of CP children.

Our own data (Wolking, Quast, and Lawton) on the Multiphasics of parents indicates that both the mothers and fathers of children diagnosed as having an organic brain syndrome were relatively more emotionally disturbed than parents of seven other nosological groups, including the mentally deficient. But the point is that all of the parents in all the groups were significantly more disturbed than adults from the general population.

There is some research evidence that sibs can be adversely affected, especially in the areas of dependency where parents expect a disproportionate amount of responsibility, usually from the oldest girl. Yet the mothers complain about the girl's moodiness and the difficulty in getting along with her when she does complain about this heavy responsibility.

The sex of the handicapped child can be an important factor in family adjustment. There seem to be more marital problems in a family as the retarded boy gets older; our society expects more from boys and parents become increasingly disappointed as social and other pressures increase.

Ordinal position can even be a significant factor since, as is the case with normal children, the eldest son often has more difficulty with the father, who is seen by him as a disciplinarian, while the mother is seen as a disciplinarian by the youngest child. Also, the normal sib of whatever age is placed in the older child role with attendant responsibilities as just mentioned. There may be some advantage if the youngest child in the family is the handicapped member—one mother recently said, "Since I have seven children, I am very thankful that Joey was the youngest, for I can put up with his being a baby longer. It would be much harder if he were the oldest, and I had to care as well for the younger children as they grew up."

The age factor is also important, since retardation means very different things at different developmental levels, a point which our chairman, Dr. Boone, has emphasized. In the early years, concern is with development—is he doing things on schedule and (especially in our culture) is he talking on schedule? Grandparents are prone to harass mothers if the child is not doing what he should for his age. It reminds me of a cartoon— I'm not much of a Gesell man concerning the very tight schedule the children are supposed to adhere to. This cartoon is of two six-year-olds sitting on a couch reading Gesell themselves. One is saying to the other, "Boy, if they're having trouble with us this year, we're going to be hellers next year."

Later in the school years, academic achievement seems to be the bugaboo which unquestionably presents the most difficult hurdle for many families in our culture. Later, the problems of ultimate adult vocation and school adjustment come to the fore. As in all our families, some parents are better able to cope with infants and the very young; other children are better during the school years, and still others are more helpful as they become young adults. This is dramatic, even in comparing spouses—maybe it is a happy circumstance for all of us that mothers tend to balance off fathers in strengths and weaknesses.

Prevalence rates of mental retardation indicate the *severely* retarded are recognized early in life. Later in childhood, especially as children reach school age, the *moderately* retarded are often identified as early as their first encounter with school and competition. Still later, in school, as work becomes harder or when life stresses become greater, the *mildly* retarded show up. This group represents some of the more difficult problems for those who are "in-betweeners"—they themselves recognize they are not as bright as their age mates, but also realize they are brighter than the more easily recognized slow child. With increasing numbers of school psychologists, and attention to the problem in general, these children are being identified in growing numbers. Unfortunately, in many communities where the

IQ is above average, the problems are even accentuated. Rather than trying to document the effects on parents of a handicapped child, emphasis will be placed on the direct clinical teaching parents have afforded us.

Procedurally, it is wise to test the child before detailed interview of the parents, partly in order to get an unbiased view of the child. With preschoolers, we often invite parents to sit in on the examination. This has the obvious advantage of seeing parent and child together. It also provides a point of reference for the parent in later discussions about strengths and weaknesses—much as the Vineland Maturity Scale offers a sort of a structured interview which parents can elaborate to help one on various points.

Having a parent sit in is a very helpful procedure even with older retarded children, especially in the case of a sensory handicapped child where the mother is probably the best "interpreter." I recently tested a seventeen-year-old multihandicapped, retarded, deaf, diabetic, seizure patient where I could not have decoded what the girl was saying without the mother present. With her I got a reliable test. Recently, I saw a thirteen-year-old retarded child who, according to history, had never been tested because he was "uncooperative, hyperactive and just fearful." It readily became apparent that the child was gradually slowing down as I talked to the mother; with studied neglect, I ignored him. Periodically, he was literally hanging on to his mother to be sure she was still there. I quickly got out a Binet kit as I talked with her, and was able to test this child, with the mother (after a while) absolutely out of his visual field in the back of the room. Obviously, I urge this as a method of getting to some children one cannot otherwise test.

In order to talk intelligently with parents, some "diagnosis" of them and of family functioning in general is necessary. Perhaps I differ with Dr. Ross here, in that I find it mandatory to know how the child came to be what he is. In other words, I go as far as diagnosing parents. Routinely in our clinic we require parents to take the Multiphasic, for example. Interestingly, we have had no trouble whatsoever with this procedure. We must now have over 2,000 sets of parents' tests. Only one parent has ever objected to this, and she said, "I know I'm incriminating myself by not taking the test," but ultimately she did take it. In some settings, a detailed social history is available, but in many cases and perhaps in the majority of situations (especially where the problem is first encountered or first presented) social data is sketchy at best. It is therefore necessary to interview parents in considerable detail, so they may learn about themselves and, also, to obtain a diagnostic aid in finding out about the child.

If a social history is available, time is profitably spent in elaborating salient leads appearing in the history.

Recently, in a continuing education course neurologically oriented for pediatricians, Leon Eisenberg (a child psychiatrist at Johns Hopkins and a scholar in the Kanner tradition) suggested that pediatricians put down their rubber hammers long enough to listen to mothers and to school people in their descriptions of behavior. He said, "The diagnosis of brain damage is a social phenomenon." What he means, obviously, is that there is valid data coming from reports of various kinds of people. In contrast to listening to parents, I have been impressed, for example, with how readily the professional person doubts reports of hyperactivity based on a fifty-minute or less one-to-one office visit. In a recent study at Kenny Rehabilitation Institute, it was found that several simple questions put to parents were of as much diagnostic value as an EEG, or a neurological examination in differentiating brain-injured from non-brain-injured children. These questions were: *Was the labor longer than usual? Is he clumsy? Is he particularly careful in trying not to make mistakes? Is he afraid of strange people?*

The following vignette shows how often parental anxiety is a factor to be dealt with; how it can be elicited in interview; how far back the antecedents of parental anxiety may go and how important this anxiety can be in the resolution of the problem presented by the child. The mother of a boy who had suffered trauma to the head as a result of an auto accident and was having learning problems in school, related she had been early sensitized to the problem of damage to the brain; she had had a younger sister who was a CP for whom this mother was responsible. Only through detailed interview with the mother did it come to light that even early in her pregnancy with this boy she was very apprehensive. I quote a letter which she volunteered later. You don't often get letters; you hear about the bad ones, but not very often do they respond in letter form. She said:

> I wish to thank you and Dr. S. for the completeness of the information given us. As is obvious from the seven-year lapse in testing done on Todd, we had adopted a "hope-for-the-best" attitude. However, with things going generally well and at the suggestion of a new pediatrician, Dr. K., we felt we should be "certain" of the future. I felt I could better face that which I undertsood rather than living with a half-fear in the background. Ironically enough, this perhaps stems from the training given me during "natural childbirth" classes and the thoroughness of the information shared with me by my obstetrician, Dr. B. The "natural childbirth" method had been selected for all my children with the thought that I would do my part in preventing brain damage or birth injuries—as had been sustained by my sister.

Now, can you imagine going into labor with that motivation? A check with the OB man, who, incidentally, became a psychiatrist, indicated he was never aware of this mother's concern —that she had never confided this to him, that even during the process he was not aware of this attitude, and he is a very astute man. It shows how these people retain this until it comes out later. It is an irony of fate that this boy in fact did suffer trauma to the head. Indicative of her current anxiety, she was attending a lecture on brain damage the day the child was brought by her husband for testing. The boy, interestingly (despite relatively minor academic problems for the insult he had sustained) was doing remarkably well. The major problem here was the mother's apprehension. In a more positive vein later in her letter the mother said:

> Perhaps I have the advantage of having my sister, and am more alert than another parent to realizing that you must remember there are other children in the family who, while sympathetic, have very important lives to lead also. Sometimes the saddened parent will feel guilty in encouraging a more gifted child because it is something the special child can never achieve.

Anyway, interviews with this mother have helped her realize her own basic training in apprehension about these problems. She has been able to modify her behavior toward her son, since she is focusing more on herself, rather than on the boy, at this stage.

It is often not easy to get the father in for interview; perhaps, because many of us are males, we tend to rationalize his claimed inability to be present. In rural Minnesota the corn has to be picked or planted—there's always a good excuse for not coming in to the hospital. My analogy often is that if the child is under an oxygen tent, the corn can wait—the father is sitting right beside the bed. We contribute to his not coming by our own attitude. We let the parents slip off the hook too easily, we rationalize all kinds of things not to involve them; all of it is of our own doing. We should be very adamant about the contribution we are making, and as Dr. Ross said the other day, it takes time—these are lifetime problems which can be averted. We should insist both parents be present.

One of our mothers of a retarded child gave us the following guide lines which she later published (Patterson, L. L. 1956):

1. Tell us the nature of our problem as soon as possible.
2. Always see both parents.
3. Watch your language [she means here, in part, not to use psychologese].
4. Help us see this is OUR problem [and what she means here is to point out that the parents have the ultimate responsibility].
5. Help us understand our problem.
6. Know your resources.
7. Never put us on the defensive.
8. Remember that parents of retarded children are just people. [Here she means don't expect too much too soon.]
9. Remember that we are parents and that you are the professional. [And here she wants us to allow parents their quota of concern and anxiety.]
10. Remember the importance of your attitude toward us.

Now, I shall try to highlight in rank order, in terms of the frequency of occurrence, factors which are significant barriers to the resolution of the problems presented by having a retarded child usually (but not necessarily) living in the home.

If these seem obvious, it may be they are so obvious that they are neglected and taken for granted. Currently, one of our staff pediatricians is doing some research on parents' questions generally on mental health which pediatricians claim they routinely answer. He is finding, for example, in the area of sex education, personal experience and opinions are given rather than facts. The factors we will consider are these:

Parents give indication that emotional or psychodynamic factors in family organization have been left unresolved.

Parents are confused because of a variety of opinions and suggestions for management.

There is lack of agreement between parents as to severity, management goals, future, etc.

Parents are in poor communication with schools and social agencies.

Parents have difficulty in knowing where to turn for advice about what appear to be simple day-to-day management problems.

To elaborate each briefly:

The first factor is the lack of dealing with parents' emotions especially the lack of awareness on the part of the husband on how much emotional and physical strain the wife is under. In-laws and relatives blame the mother for not being able to manage the child, and label her as inadequate or unfeeling. If the husband is not supportive, the wife becomes hostile, creating situations which will require him then to be more helpful, and this ends up only in further estrangement. There is a popular gimmick some wives use—they simply refuse to get a driver's license, complaining that for some reason they simply can't learn to drive a car. Obviously, this puts the husband in the position of having to be responsible for all transportation problems.

The unrelenting constancy of care is a problem—often, out of guilt, the mother feels no one but herself can care for the child. The consequence is no baby sitters and no social life. This is especially true, I think, for young married couples where the role-shift is rapid; from fiance, to wife, to mother and then, especially, if the first child is retarded. Reuben Hill, in our Family Life Division at the University, has some very interesting data on the importance of this role change which perhaps has not had sufficient attention. The problem is further compounded if there is a financial strife, or the husband is devoting all his energies to his work. For example, in our hospital there is what we call a "resident" syndrome where the patient is brought as the problem, but the main problem is the father's abrogation of his parental responsibility, of the father and even the husband role. This is not limited to medical residents, obviously. This happens in all walks of life. Often mothers in our insular society have no Aunt Jenny or any confidant at all to whom to turn. It is sometimes wise to encourage these mothers to seek some part-time help or even conscientiously seek a program of activity outside the home. Obviously, this can be sabotaged if the husband is not in accord.

Often the constancy of care problem is of the mother's own making. I think she tends to overidentify with the retarded or handicapped child, especially in his being rejected in so many ways. Being rejected, he turns to her, his dependency is then reciprocated, and a symbiotic relationship develops. This is not unlike pathologic dependency in other kinds of problems—for example, in the so-called school phobic child, where the primary problem is the separation anxiety generated by the mother's own unresolved dependency. We have had cases in our hospital where the mother had to be hospitalized when the child was hospitalized because of this very close interdependency relationship. This circular dependency can drastically limit the social life of the entire family and especially the love relationship between the husband and wife. The problem can be even more complicated in the case of a child with cerebral dysfunction, since this dependency in these children is harder to weigh. In some cases, to use Dabrowski's term, a positive disintegration occurs (i.e., the dependency can be functional). I recently had a thirteen-year-old girl whose mother was irritated because the child would hang onto her, and the mother would say, "Now, you're a big girl." For example, as they would be walking downtown, the mother would say, "Don't keep grabbing onto me; walk by yourself." Come to find out this girl literally did not know her left from her right. Under the pressure of downtown traffic, she would just as readily jump into the path of a vehicle as away from it. When this was learned, then the mother understood this kind of dependency was functional for this person. It is hard for the parents to judge how much of it is par and how much of it they should not encourage.

Sometimes, even the sexual compatability of the parents can be affected by having a handicapped child. There was recently an old movie on television titled, "Light in the Piazza," the story of a beautiful but retarded daugther and the problems of getting her married. Dramatically, when the husband flew to meet his family in Italy, greeted his wife and made some overtures to her, she started to cry. She was so preoccupied with the daughter that he said, "Are you going to continue forever being a guardian to her or are you also going to be a wife to me?" He left in a huff. This is a very real problem.

The variety of ways in which parental emotional involvement can occur is endless; one has to make guesses. One has to stick his neck out and make some guesses as to what is going on in the family. Only by making some assumptions and testing them out is it possible to find out what is going on. Many professionals, for some reason, don't want to level with parents. This occurs in many disciplines. Just the other day I learned of a social worker of whom a mother said, "Well, my husband started to cry and so the social worker quickly changed the subject." They never did get to the problem of why the man was crying, and skirted around the whole problem.

A *second factor* is that parents are barraged from a great many sources with varying information and opinions. It is very necessary for us to know accurately what the medical condition is, what they have been told and when. We also need to have some sort of contract with them as we do in psychotherapy, i.e. find out what they want to know—who is hurting—before any interpretation we might make is inopportunely imposed. This is especially necessary in the case of a child with cerebral dysfunction, where, even if the diagnosis is made, this may not be the problem at all—the mother's anxiety may be the central problem.

Parents are unclear about prediction and what the future holds. More often than not, they think the retardate will catch up. Yet, on the other hand, they are many times more pessimistic about the ultimate future of the child than is warranted.

Too often predictions have been made from early data to terminal adult level with no scientific basis. Parents are unclear about employability of certain IQ levels, what special classes are all about, and have very little information about institutions. In some cases, often iatrogenic, parents have been advised to keep searching, with the implication, "Just do the best you can, something will happen." This is an invitation to shop. Parents are sometimes shocked to be told nothing can be done medically to alter the condition, but that their energies are better spent in coping with behavior.

It is wise in most cases to be conservative in making predictions. In the early years, it is safe to predict about two years at a time, then having the patient return for more definitive examination up until school age.

I have been following one child, first seen at the age of four when her IQ was 58; at age eight her IQ was 78 and at age fourteen her IQ was 116—exactly doubled in ten years. Her clinical picture at four seemed a relatively classically retarded child; in the next examination she appeared to be a child with cerebral dysfunction. Now, in teen age, she is diagnosed as schizophrenic. So, here again, is another compounding factor. Incidentally, everybody agrees that whatever she has, her mental illness seems to be organically based.

In the case of children with cerebral dysfunction, we have been impressed with the increasing frequency of their having early Binets in the low average range—for example, at age five where they first start school—to find later, at age ten, an appreciably lower IQ. This could be, in part, a function of scatter; more commonly than not a function of scatter as the child gets older. I tested a child the other day with a verbal-performance discrepancy of 50 points—a verbal IQ of 70 and a performance

IQ of 120. There have been some cases like this which we've followed and found to become very productive people with excellent employment records. Jean Holroyd (1965) has some interesting data on this—her criterion is a 25-point discrepancy and especially with a lowered performance, finds a high relationship with central nervous system involvement.

Generally, in problems of prediction, a happier milieu is provided when both family and child must cope with only one time segment at a time. Certainly, there are sufficient maturational changes over time, especially in the early years, to justify this approach. This philosophy holds even through the school years, especially since children with cerebral dysfunction do change and mature in certain channels, enough to alter their life style drastically. One child following encephalitis can be retarded for the rest of his life, while another, seemingly equally traumatized, may recover with minimal residual.

Often parents have been given a variety of opinions, or in some cases have grossly distorted what they have been told, or have been so emotionally upset they did not hear what they were told. Because of any or all of these, they are likely to approach a new person defensively, if not with some hostility, and will even hide factual information defensively. They are astute at using the professional as a scapegoat, and so we have to be alerted to this and not retaliate in kind. This is very common with students who find they get angry at a parent who is needling them, and do not permit the parent to have this defensiveness.

Then, again, parents have accused professionals of giving them suggestions unrealistic for a particular family. In the same vein, a parent coming with a specific practical question will find it parried with generalizations and theory. Some professionals simply do not have the answers but in this case several alternative solutions might be offered. If these are based on another family's experience, it doesn't sound so much like a professional opinion. Parents have also complained they were led to believe that recommendations for changing behavior would result in quick solutions. This, unfortunately, is not

usually true—adjustment, for example, to special classes sometimes takes years.

A *third factor is* lack of agreement between parents as to
severity or true nature of the problem. Often, parents have never
reached the point of being really able to discuss the child, or
their feelings about the child, with each other in any kind of
intimacy. They always skirt it. It seems amazing the number
of times parents have said, "Not until we sat in front of you
did we really ever discuss this between us." Obviously, mothers
feel especially guilty that it was something they did when they
were carrying the child and feel this is their cross to bear.
Mothers seem to feel very guilty for many reasons.

The resistance so often referred to of parents being unwill-
ing or unable to accept the idea of their child's retardation or
defect is recognized by most workers as being emotionally based.
One must be alerted to the idiosyncratic twists this can
take. For example, it is not uncommon to find parents of a
retarded or brain-injured child making a case for his being
neurotic or even psychotic. Some parents (in their judgment)
would rather have the child schizophrenic because they think
the child is then more amenable to change; yet people will
blame them for having such an attitude.

An initial buffer item to lead into this problem of parental
agreement is to routinely ask each parent independently to
estimate the mental age of the child. "Your child is six by his
birth date. Compared with your other children when they
were six, what is he doing for his age?" To me, it's striking to
see the accuracy with which parents who are objective can
predict. It takes me two or three hours of testing, but they will
hit this mental age right on the head. On the other hand, if
they are emotionally involved, the converse holds—their estimates
are way off.

A *fourth factor is that* school or other agency and the parents
are in a bind. There is a need for on-going case work or
counseling which is simply not being fulfilled. This is a chronic
problem, especially in the lower SES classes where they do not
understand the nature of special classes, the potential of the

child and many other problems. They, for example, feel the child will be unhappy at being segregated in a special class. Parents do not realize that when a child has to be moved, in the beginning he complains, but in more cases than not, after he is in there, he is very much relieved not to be low man on the totem pole all the time—in fact, is happy to be top dog for a change. The children themselves have expressed relief at not having to compete at levels on which they cannot compete.

The problem of semantics is especially important. I had one mother who was in a hassle with both the schools and the social agency over her misunderstanding of the terms alone. She said, "My child is not mentally retarded like they keep telling me." I simply said, "What do you mean by mental retardation?" She meant mental illness. She said, "Oh, I know he is slow, but he is not mentally retarded." So, no one had ever taken the time to decode what she was saying, but assumed she was not "accepting."

Another mother had been told by teachers for three successive years that her child was immature, but no one had ever delineated the meaning, let alone the degree. Ironically, the mother said to me, "I know the child is retarded; why didn't they say so?"

Another mother of a three-and-one-half-year-old child was told the child was "socially immature" in nursery school. The mother was flabbergasted and asked when *could* a child be socially immature, if it wasn't at three-and-one-half? The teacher knew what *she meant;* that the child was not behaving like others of that age; but she had not communicated this to the parent.

As a consultant to public schools and to a service project in a city hospital, I see these problems *in situ*. It seems to me the pediatrician often is either not interested in the area of the parent counseling, or feels he is incompetent, or just will not take the time. The time factor is a tremendously important item here. School personnel, even psychologists and counselors, seem insecure and unsure as to the depth they dare go in working with such problems. There is even national controversy regarding psychological intervention in family problems as a proper role for schools. Tom Szasz (1964) has an excellent article in which he feels psychiatry should be divorced from education—just as separate as church from state, with which I do not agree at all. It simply doesn't work. Communication is difficult enough even within one functional unit. This whole business of teams is difficult at best. The point is if this is attempted across agencies, the families end up as the losers.

There is a great need to involve the family and the community more deeply with these problems, since it is likely that the manipulation of the environment is going to ameliorate these problems more than direct work, of whatever nature, with the child.

Child neurologists are, for example, telling parents, at least in our hospital, that they would rather try psychological methods of modifying behavior before embarking on an empirical drug control approach.

Shakespeare said, "The fault, Dear Brutus, is not in our stars, But in ourselves, that we are underlings." I don't agree with him, since these concepts are steeped in deep historical roots in philosophy, are unidimensional and ignore the large influence of the environment. The recent upsurge of interest in behavior modification through operant conditioning would seem to offer great promise for the family and community management of handicapped children. To quote Gerald Patterson (1965) from Oregon, in a paper on the *modification of hyperactive behavior in children:* "I would hazard a guess that ten years from now, most of our efforts will be directed toward changing the reinforcement schedules provided by the social environment rather than attempting to manipulate directly the behavior of the child. (Paper read at SRCD convention in Minneapolis in 1965.)

To show the extent to which a hyperactive child can disrupt family living, I recently had a three-and-a-half-year-old boy who, in addition to being hyperkinetic, slept very poorly, if at all. He first insisted on coming into the parents' bedroom; he then insisted on coming into bed with them; and currently he is sleeping on top of their bodies, if you can imagine—he insists on this. There is little doubt in this case that there may be an organic component in this child's behavior. Obviously, the wrong kind of conditioning the parents are providing has placed them in their present dilemma. For a solution to this problem, again I would refer you to the excellent work being done by Gerald Patterson. He has some cookbook-type operations to deal with problems like this.

A *fifth factor is the parental problem of* where to turn for day-to-day ongoing help with relatively simple problems of management. To whom can the mother turn when her child is pulling up the neighbor's tulips, or drinking ink? We professionals as a group are not sufficiently appreciative of the very practical and difficult problems these parents face with a hyperactive child, for example.

For many mothers, it is difficult for them to learn they cannot assume that ordinary verbal instructions, for example, will be comprehended and followed. I recently had a very difficult differential diagnostic problem in a four-and-a-half-year-old boy who turned out to be aphasic. He came from a bilingual home and was thought to be retarded or emotionally disturbed; his not understanding or talking was attributed to the bilingual aspect. To make a long story short, these parents were in psychotherapy for two years, based largely on the mother's inability to communicate with this child. It's a tragedy these parents were divorced recently, primarily on the basis of the husband's not supporting his wife; everyone was blaming her for the management of the child. She had never known a condition such as aphasia *per se* could exist, and simply did not understand that this boy was not even clear about right and wrong, or yes and no. Unfortunately, the husband was the most unsympathetic of anyone.

Mothers of normal youngsters for years have been eager for a "cookbook" on child-rearing. Only recently has there been a Spock on nonmedical help. Mothers of handicapped children are in a double bind. In-laws are unsympathetic or many professionals don't take the time. Often, caseworkers assigned to MR units either have too big a case load or are too young and too inexperienced. In any event, they don't seem to be adequately trained to cope with these problems. The unfortunate part is that these problems are not of sufficient magnitude to be classed as psychiatric problems, so, for example, they don't get professional help through the existing mental health centers.

One source of help that seems especially effective are mothers' clubs, which meet on an informal basis for group discussions led by a variety of professionals. In our hospital, we are experimenting with such meetings, dealing with a variety of problems. In heart disease, for example, there is a group of parents whose children come to our hospital from all over the world for heart operations. These children would come into the hospital perfectly happy, but after a short stay there, would start all kinds of problems on the ward. It became readily apparent they were simply responding to the parental anxiety before the heart surgery—that they were simply a direct expression of the parents' anxiety. All we did was to talk with these parents, not about the heart, but about their feelings concerning the pending operation. This is very helpful in management of the children.

Obviously, the existing parent groups, such as the National Association for Brain Injured and similar state organizations are very helpful, since historically, parents have, for the most part, helped each other. Perhaps this is one of the best sources— to train parents to help each other, and may be ultimately a very feasible attack on this problem.

Sidney Bijou, in Illinois (whose work has been mentioned in other contexts) is doing some most provocative work in shaping the behavior of parents through experiments working directly with the reinforcement techniques parents use. Bijou simply conditions them in their operations with the children. Similar operant conditioning techniques have been shown to be equally effective with classroom teachers, and there seems little doubt that research in this area is bound to be fruitful.

While we in a teaching hospital cannot provide ongoing service, after a diagnostic study and an interpretive planning workup, we do ask parents to return in three months for some feedback. This serves the double function of clarifying what was discussed by having the parents go over what they understood, and additionally, checking on the efficacy of whatever plans were made.

In summary, until such time when there are more centralized

agencies providing ongoing contact, it would behoove any of us who diagnose, treat or recommend treatment to spend equal time and energy with the parents as with the child. Steps should be taken to increase agreement between parents intellectually and emotionally on their values pertaining to the handicapped child and the family in general. We should watch our language. There should be an awareness that the future adjustment of the older normal sibs may be affected if they are given too much responsibility. The role and responsibilities of the father should be emphasized—especially in order to minimize the mother-child interdependency.

REFERENCES

1. BLODGETT, H. E., AND WARFIELD, G. J.: *Understanding Mentally Retarded Children.* New York, Appleton, 1959.
2. FARBER, B.: Effects of a severely retarded child on family integration. *Monogr Soc Res Child Develop, 24,* 1959.
3. FARBER, B.: Family organization and crisis: Maintenance of integration in families with a severely mentally retarded child. *Monogr Soc Res Child Develop, 25,* 1960.
4. HOLROYD, J., AND WRIGHT, F.: Neurological implications of WISC Verbal Performance discrepancies in a psychiatric setting. *J Consult Psychol, 29,* 1965.
5. JORDAN, T. E.: *The Mentally Retarded.* Columbus, Ohio, Charles E. Merrill Books, Inc., 1961.
6. KANNER, L.: Feeblemindedness, absolute, relative and apparent, *Nerv Child, 7,* 1948.
7. PATTERSON, G. R.: The modification of hyperactive behavior in children. Paper read at SRCD Convention, Minneapolis, Minn., 1965.
8. PATTERSON, L. L.: Some pointers for professionals. *Children, 3,* 1956.
9. REYNOLDS, M. C., ELLIS, R. E., AND KILAND, J. R.: *A Study of Public School Children with Severe Mental Retardation.* Research project No. 6, State of Minnesota, Department of Education, Statistical Division, St. Paul 1, Minnesota, 1953.
10. SZASZ, T. S.: Psychiatry in public schools. *Teachers College Record, 66,* 1964.
11. WOLKING, W. D., QUAST, W., AND LAWTON, J. J., JR.: MMPI profiles of the parents of behaviorally disturbed children and parents from the general population. *J Clin Psychol, 1,* 1966.

DISCUSSION I

WILLIAM J. VON LACKUM, PH.D.

Dr. Quast has dealt with parental interaction not only in the diagnosis of children with psychological problems, but also in the problems of case management.

This speaker would like to direct one specific question to Dr. Quast. This question relates to the administration of the MMPI to both parents of children being seen in the clinic; also, to the relationship, if any, this practice has demonstrated between the profiles of the parents and the behavior of the child, or the future of clinical intervention.

Anxiety has many concomitants. The one with which we wish to deal is the extreme egocentrism which always accompanies strong dysphoric feelings.

Children, with their normal dependency needs, best mature in an environment characterized by the presence of strongly sociocentric adults. To the child with a developmental problem secondary to any type of handicap, this need is even more imperative. There are methods for dealing with anxiety, and the psychologist, along with other members of the mental health discipline, knows, or certainly should know, what they are. These methods, however, become particularly difficult to employ when the anxiety under question is within ourselves. In spite of this knowledge, however, there is a very marked tendency to deal with problems like this at a highly cognitive level.

The practicing clinician characteristically deals with the behavior of a patient in terms of the anxiety patterns which he (the patient) presents. Unfortunately, however, we do not always deal with the anxiety patterns of those who, a) inform us as to the behavior of the child, or b) those with whom we are attempting to work out long-term case-management problems. It is as though we frequently utilize all of our empathy on the child, with little, if any, left over for parents and other adults involved in the situation. It is felt that an overt, conscious recognition and treatment of this anxiety would make it much easier to apply the material which Dr. Quast has presented.

In the diagnostic aspect of the problem, concentration on the anxieties of the parents and authority figures in the child's environment should make it easier to cut through the exaggerations and sometimes overgeneralizations which these individuals are likely to demonstrate. One indication of these exaggerations is seen in the effort of the authority figures in contact with the child to arrive at a "diagnosis" rather than giving an objective description of the child's behavior. The lay diagnoses to which reference is made include such terms as "immaturity"; "attention-getting"; "he only does it to punish me"; with even such characterization as "strong-willed"; and once in a while, "he's just a plain stinker." These characterizations, of course, do not describe the behavior of the individual in question, and, thereby, are of little use to the clinician in attempting to arrive at some professional formulation. They reflect, rather, the anxiety (or the defense against this anxiety) by recourse to highly egocentric needs of these authority figures as they face the frustration presented by the inability of the child in question to live up to their expectations. This frustration leads to anxiety, forcing a type of what might be called social regression, in which the individual drops back to a highly moralistic frame of reference in an effort to cope with this problem. Anxiety on the clinician's part plays a marked role with attempts to predict such things as the child's future capacities, as seen from the standpoint of educability and employability. One resolution of this anxiety may lead to the error of extreme dogmatism. This, too, is a good defense. A second type of resolution may lead to such vagueness, that no real information is imparted at all to the important authority figures in the child's environment. Of course, the most difficult thing for the clinician to say in terms of his own anxiety is, "I frankly don't know"; even when he can hedge this situation by saying, possibly, "In six months or a year we will know," and to do this in such a way as to maintain the security of the family while the workup continues.

Now, if one applies this anxiety concept to the parents' reaction to a handicapped child, it is easily seen why the mother, with her propensity for caretaking, will tend to exaggerate the dependency needs of the child. But the father, who characteristically projects the child into the future in terms of his ability to achieve, is quite likely to take the opposite point of view, as indicated in Dr. Quast's paper.

We are also worried about what might be called "community anxiety." With the advent of the first sputnik and the ensuing "space race," a predictable widespread fear was identifiable. One manifestation of this anxiety has been a marked limitation on the normal educational dependency of all children. This is seen as grammar school children prepare "research reports," study advanced mathematics, learn to spell and classify dinosaurs, with minimum assistance from authority figures. This is all subsumed under the guise of preparing the child for a college. The emphasis for all this seems to be on long hours of preparation and independence of behavior, rather than content. Therefore, it is presumably meant, they are going to make the child just as uncomfortable in grammar school and high school as the authority figures were when they were in college.

Now, if one takes the case of the child with a cerebral dysfunction, the problem becomes more acute. What this child basically needs is an intensification and, to some extent, a prolongation of his nurturance, as he attempts to cope with his problems which (among other things) include poor attention, distractibility, and emotional lability. These are areas in which intervention and prolonged intervention of reliable authority figures are necessary. Instead of this type of support, the child will probably be subjected to some kind of ridicule, will be given a few bad names and will end up by repeating the grade he could not solve in the first place. One of the most dramatic cases of this is a child who had a tested 130 intelligence quotient on the Stanford-Binet. It was recommended this child repeat nursery school because she was not emotionally ready for kindergarten!

Along the same line, is it possible that much of the time and effort devoted to the development of independence in the mentally retarded child might not more realistically be directed towards adjusting him to a functioning dependence on more capable authority figures? In this connection, the training of a whole contingent of people who can offer sustaining support to parents and to children is an excellent suggestion. Methods for the control of these individuals' anxieties (particularly the egocentric resolution of these anxieties) must be emphasized much more than a development of specific skills. In this context, this speaker's experience in working with the Training Group Method with a group of people in part-time counseling, (a group of ministers) has been that though they have the skills and techniques, it is the anxiety problem which gives them trouble.

The question that Dr. Quast raises about family disintegration in the presence of a handicapped child is certainly worth deep consideration from this point of view. This, too, should be viewed from the standpoint of the egocentricity which develops in the face of severe anxiety as these people feel it. Mention has already been made of the conflicting resolution of anxiety patterns between husband and wife. This frequently leads to a great deal of friction in and of itself. In addition to this, there is the curtailing of opportunity for other siblings because of two reasons. The first is the financial demands of the handicapped child, particularly with a chronic handicap. The second is the increased dependency requirements which this child inevitably manifests. This curtailing is certainly not to be understood by the other children, not basically, so the result is frequently some limitation in their own self-concept formation.

It seems most families of which a handicapped child is a member, can be characterized as a group which has lost its initiative in dealing with the problems of life. These families frequently become so fatigued in efforts to cope with the day-to-day inadequacies of the child, that little energy is left for the child's constructive planning, and no energy left at all for their personal constructive planning. For example, a family (known to the speaker) had an extremely hyperkinetic, although not mentally retarded, child. At the time he came to clinical attention, the husband and wife had not been out a single night for four years since this child was born. They naturally found it difficult to obtain baby-sitters who could care for the child; when the parents could find them, the anxiety of divorcing themselves from this child for even an evening was more than they could handle. Also, they found it difficult to have guests because of the anxiety aroused by the child's constant acting up. This family was definitely headed for complete disintegration in the divorce court until a successful medical regime was established, bringing the child more in line with normal expectancies.

Consultation encouraging the parents of handicapped children to aggressively compensate for their disappointment by emphasizing opportunities for their own personal achievement, as well as constructive planning for the child himself, seems to be a most effective approach. This can best be achieved by dealing directly with these anxieties as such, as well as dealing directly with all people concerned, whether they represent the parents, the community or other authority figures in the school system and in law enforcement agencies. This will lay the best groundwork for any type of constructive behavior.

DISCUSSION II
MARY I. DUWALL, PH.D.

Dr. Quast has most adequately pointed out the many variables one must be aware of and be prepared to cope with, in an interpretative interview. This speaker will confine her discussion at the molecular level, since Dr. von Lackum has already elaborated on some of the pertinent points at the molar level.

The suggestion made that we use the term cerebral dysfunction instead of brain damage must be questioned. At least one reaction to this suggestion is: "Dr. Quast, you are playing a psychological trick on me. You are climbing higher on the abstraction ladder, saying less that is specific, and making it sound more scientific." The speaker is also reminded of the following passage from Lewis Carroll's *Alice through the Looking Glass:*

> "When *I* use a word," Humpty Dumpty said, in a rather scornful tone, "it means just what I choose it to mean—neither more nor less."
>
> "The question is," said Alice, "whether you *can* make words mean so many different things."
>
> "The question is," said Humpty Dumpty, "which is to be master— that's all."

In using this quotation, a question might be raised which the panel[1] will possibly discuss, since each seems to have an idiosyncratic understanding of the word "brain damage" in terms of prognosis, behavioral manifestations, the importance of diagnosis, and the organic-functional issue. Dr. Quast has said he does not wish to raise this old organic-functional issue, but he has raised it in his suggested change of terminology.

Apparently, psychologists, pediatricians, and neurologists get together in a particular location and learn to share a common language. This investigator polled her associates as to their interpretation of the words "brain damage" and "cerebral dysfunction." Some interesting and negative reactions to the term "cerebral dysfunction" were received. This interviewer was told she was impyling that the brain was structurally intact, that this term excluded the cerebellum and included psychosis. Some of the respondents implied she was being vague and evading the issue.

The global term "brain damage" really is not that much better, because it is also vague. However, through widespread usage, it has become an accepted term. Why not refine this term for greater communicative value?

Another comment concerns the hyperactive, or the hyperkinetic, child. These terms are applied to a large, undifferentiated group of children; limited recognition is given to the different types of children falling into this group. Perhaps the results obtained from the methods we use are more related to our ability to identify the children who will respond to a particular method, than to the superiority of one approach over the other. Psychological methods produce good results with some children, but with other children it appears medication is required. We have been finding there are usually good results from medication, if there is unanimous agreement among staff members that the child would benefit from medication. When there is disagreement, usually we do not get good results with medication.

Perhaps we should expend some effort in improving our

---

[1]The panel here refers to Drs. A. Barclay, Wallace A. Kennedy, Henry Leland, Wentworth Quast, Ralph M. Reitan, and Alan O. Ross. Moderator was Dr. Nelms B. Boone.

skills to recognize the qualitative differences in the behavior of hyperactive children who respond to medication, and those who do not. Using a multidisciplinary approach, it would be possible to develop criteria enabling us to classify types of hyperactivity in children. When this has been done, we will then be ready to determine the merit of different approaches for treatment of the hyperactive child.

DISCUSSION III
Charles P. DeMinico, M.D.

It might be useful to present some specific examples of useful methods to ease anxiety in parents of children with mental retardation or organic brain disorders. The need to bring comfort to these people in their distress during the course of a workup cannot be overlooked.

Interviews with these parents involve no specific structure or planned format. They are allowed to talk and express their feelings, with a little guidance as needed. During the discussion, various areas of parental concern are usually elicited easily. Although the psychiatrist's function is primarily a diagnostic or evaluative one, some time is reserved towards the end of the interview for explanation or clarification. This must be done in a way that does not interfere with the team approach. At the Child Development Center of the University of Tennessee, where this speaker has been a consultant, the results of interviews from the various team members are collated into a final summary and presented to the parents at the last *informing interview*. To avoid interfering with this team approach, one must be careful about offering premature advice or reassurance. Some examples of how this can be attained safely in such a settling will be presented:

> *One situation occurs* when the investigation might have been in progress for six months to a year, with the parents becoming impatient and a little agitated about the fleeting time, and what is being done as a result of the multiple visits they have made to the clinic. In such cases, it is explained that the time delay was not accidental, but has actually been a purposeful part of the study. This gives the staff members a better picture of the problem, and

affords a longitudinal view of the child as he progresses over a period of time. This point of view pleases a good number of parents because of the common complaint stated resentfully, such as: "How could Dr. X have been sure that my child was retarded after seeing him only once or twice in his office?" has often been heard.

Another function is occasional cautious reassurance, but only if the results are obvious. This is done when parents have a specific vague fear or premonition of what the investigation might uncover, (e.g. retardation, brain damage, hereditary factors). In such a case, it is obvious from the workup preceding the interview that there is no problem along this specific line. For instance, when there is a learning difficulty in the presence of a normal IQ, something as follows might be said: "One thing I can tell you; our tests so far show there is no mental retardation."

Another method by which the parents can be comforted is in the "softening" of concepts they have already gathered from other clinics or doctors or from their readings. For example, they might have heard the term "brain damage" used to describe a perceptual motor incoordination which may have been determined by the performance of various psychological tests (such as the Bender Visual Motor Gestalt Test). In such cases, one may try to mitigate fantasies which the parents might have conjured from the use of word "damage" as a picture of a brain with a "hole" in it. To dilute this harsh word, a spectrum concept is used of the various ranges of normal functioning (i.e. from awkwardness on one end of the scale to professional skill on the other end). An individual (in this case a psychiatrist) could use himself as an example of being pretty dumb as compared to Einstein, Werner von Braun, Pablo Casals, yet it doesn't prevent him from making a living in an area outside of these specialized fields. This does not mean the existence of a problem is denied when it is there. It is not necessary to resort to the ostrich concept; at the same time we need not paint a black picture in the presence of minimum or moderate disability.

This leads to something which has been of concern for several years and which Dr. Quast has mentioned in his presentation: namely, our use of the expression "brain damage." There must be a term somewhere in our behavioral, medical, or neurological vocabulary preventing the image in the minds of parents depicting something shattered, crushed or smashed as synonymous with the word "damaged." The term "brain injury" was used because it sounded more hopeful (e.g. a mental picture could be painted of a fractured leg mending in the cast [i.e. injured] as contrasted with a smashed leg which will never function as a useful limb [i.e. damaged]). However, even this term is a poor substitute, and it has backfired at times. We should reserve the expression "brain damage" for the obviously gross or microscopic brain cell or tissue defect appearing in the effects of severe trauma, infection, or congenital defect, with measurable neurological deficit elicited by clinical examination (impaired reflexes, tremors, or adiadokokinesis). The other cerebral dysfunctions manifested by relatively simple behavioral phenomena (hyperactivity and distractibility, a reading disability, and other specific disabilities) should avoid the "damaged" label with all its implications.

Some of the difficulties encountered with the term "brain damage" (even in cases with impaired neurological function) can be exemplified by notes from the following case histories:

Case 1: Sue is an adopted twelve-year-old girl who is described by her mother as "defiant, disobedient, uncommunicative, impertinent, sullen." The mother is a rather intolerant, rigid, compulsive, hypercritical, and overconscientious middle-aged woman. A previous study at a children's diagnostic center presented the mother with a diagnosis of "chronic brain syndrome" on the basis of psychological tests. Neurological examination showed a "certain amount of fine difficulties in coordination, more particularly evident in complex performances and drawings." EEG revealed a "hypothalamic dysrhythmia." The mother's understanding of the child's problem was as follows: "Dr. V (neurosurgeon) told me that Sue has severe brain damage, a convulsive type . . ." On the first interview the child was asked what her problem was, and she replied, "My brain is damaged —mother told me." With that said, it is not necessary to go into the dynamics of the feelings this adopted mother harbors for this girl.

Case 2: Mrs. W. is a thirty-year-old married woman, mother of two boys. Her nine-year-old son was studied at a children's clinic and labeled "brain damaged." The boy's IQ was in the 130's; the Bender was distorted in a typically organic pattern; EEG revealed "cerebral dysrhythmia." A neurological examination was performed, and no positive pathological findings were reported. However, the examiner performed an EEG on the mother, and the findings were similar to those noted in her son's study. This suggested to the examiner "a genetical and probably familial basis for his personality disorder." The mother was referred for depression; she presented herself as "unworthy as a wife, mother and human being—I have failed miserably." She had been told about the coincidental findings on the electroencephalograms, and their similarities to each other. She was ambivalent towards her alcoholic father, and dreaded hereditary traits he might have passed on to her; she mentioned this often in her interviews. On her fifth visit, with reference to her attitude towards her son, she described him as "a worthless baby out of a worthless mother." It was interesting to note that a comprehensive social history taken at the referring diagnostic center revealed the boy had been delivered by Caesarean section as an emergency due to "foetal distress." Also, at age five, in a fall from a bicycle, he had suffered a skull fracture, resulting in unconsciousness and subsequent disorientation. These possibilities as part of the etiological basis for the son's troubles were overlooked when this guilt-ridden mother was presented with her "genetic counseling."

These parents present themselves to us with a complex of problems. Their children have problems which we want to help solve, and other family members have problems related to the basic complaint. We would do well to avoid complicating matters with scary words and frightening concepts.

VIII

PROBLEMS IN EVALUATION OF
RESIDUAL EFFECTS OF HEAD INJURY

Ray W. Mackey, M.D.

T HE INCREASING number of motor vehicle accidents with resultant brain injury, and the increasing number of litigations
on behalf of injured individuals, create a major problem for the
clinician and psychologist in attempting to determine residual
CNS effects. Patients and their representatives are inclined to
give undue emphasis to transitory effects such as nervousness,
inability to concentrate, headaches, and vasomotor symptoms.
But the clinician, in an effort not to be misled by these subjective factors, tends to consider only gross neurological and
psychological deficit as a definitive organic sequelae. The latter
viewpoint, which is essentially *res ipsa loquitur,* is probably more
valid since it automatically excludes the transient effects of
head injury, and those complaints focused on by litigation-
conscious patients and attorneys on minor head injuries. However, it does seem likely that such an approach overlooks some
significant impairments.

The studies of Russell (1932) and Smith (1961) have indicated that the length of the coma and the post-traumatic
amnesia following head injury have a direct relationship to the
extent of cerebral injury, and thus, to prognosis. Their studies
show a useful method of classifying head injury:

Slight Concussion . . .	Transient disturbance of consciousness PTA under one hour
Moderate Concussion . .	Transient disturbance of consciousness PTA 1-24 hours
Severe Concussion . . .	Delayed recovery of consciousness PTA 1-7 days
Very Severe Concussion .	Prolonged coma or stupor PTA over 7 days.

186

The period of post-traumatic amnesia is that time during which the patient lacks the capacity to store memory of current events. Their studies indicate that the duration of PTA increases with age (in adults). Also ". . . of about 100 different signs and symptoms, PTA is the most sensitive and reliable index of severity for cases without signs of focal damage, such as depressed fracture of intracranial hemorrhage."

With reference to children, several studies (Rowbotham 1954, Dillon and Leopold, 1961), have commented on behavioral and personality changes such as nervousness, bad temper, aggressive or antisocial behavior. Headaches and dizziness, although present as a postconcussion symptom, seem to be less prominent than in adults.

After a detailed analysis of ten cases with very severe concussion, Richardson concluded such injuries were likely to be followed by memory defects which interfere with academic and social adjustment: ". . . The estimated moderate loss of points on formal intelligence tests (10 to 20 points) in no way represents the long-term crippling effects of the injury on the patient and family." He comments on the prevalence of wide range in various intellectual abilities; poor rote memory; academic difficulties in the classroom, such as distractibility; poor comprehension, perseverance, which were not previously present; major changes in behavior, and tendency for neurological findings (in some patients) to show some gradual improvement for as long as three years.

It has long been postulated that the mechanical effects of acceleration and deceleration on a semisolid organ such as the brain were capable of producing organic injury to the brain, but pathological confirmation has been lacking. In 1956, Strich demonstrated wide-spread, diffuse white-matter degeneration in patients manifesting severe dementia and neurological deficit subsequent to head injury. Again (1961) he reported additional cases with histologic evidence, supporting the idea that shearing of nerve fibers produces the damaging effect. It has previously been suggested that alterations in neural protein subserve the memory process. The Watson-Crick model of the macromolecule DNA (presented in 1953) has provided a molecular explanation for the template needed, not only for genetic transmission, but also, for possible storage and preservation of memory. Hyden (1960) postulated that cytoplasmic RNA may be specified by glialneural excitation. This specific RNA provides a template for specific amino acid sequences in protein production; dissociation of this specific protein is capable of inducing activity in transmitter substances (RNA) and postsynaptic excitation.

An interesting speculation related to this topic concerns the question whether local cerebral trauma sustained at an early age produces the same type of psychological deficits as that produced by similar injury in an adult. Russell (1948) has proposed that because of the conditioning effect of the prefrontal area on the left temporoparietal region during early life, injury to the prefrontal region in young children should produce a more diffuse, nonspecific intellectual deficit. Clinical experience tends to support this hypothesis, but difficulties in proving it are obvious. Oldfield and Williams (1961) have presented a case report of extensive clinical and psychological follow-up on a man who suffered a penetrating injury to the right prefrontal area as an infant of five and one-half months. The impression at age eighteen years was that of low-grade mentality with mild behavior disorder. There was no special difficulty in abstraction and use of categories, as has been previously reported with frontal lobe damage in adults.

The following two case reports are illustrative of some of the difficulties in evaluation of head injuries.

CASE 1: W. D., a fourteen-year-old white male, was first seen for examination on February 1, 1962. His history indicated incidence of a head injury and bilateral leg fractures in an auto-pedestrian accident. By history, there had been local injury and contusion in the right occipital region of the skull with associated coma, convulsions; a subdural collection of blood had been removed via burr holes. Specific information regarding the duration of depressed consciousness is not available, but he apparently was comatose for at least one day, and the post-traumatic amensia was greater than seven days. Post-traumatic residuals included mental confusion, visual difficulties, and some left-sided weakness with gradual clearing over several months.

The current difficulties at the time first seen were mainly concerned with poor progress in school work. He was having difficulties mainly with poor retention and recall, as exemplified by inability to remember assignments; his ability to learn appeared to his parents to be not as good as during the year prior to his injury. He was receiving Dilantin 90 mg tid prescribed prophylactically by his neurosurgeon. Positive findings included surgical burr holes in the right temporal and both occipital regions, injury scars on the left knee and right lumbar region. Cranial nerve examination was normal except for a trace of nystagmus, thought to be due to Dilantin. There was no detectable motor deficit in strength or coordination. All the deep tendon reflexes were brisk with unsustained ankle clonus and mild hypertonicity in the legs. A mild lateralized increase of DTR in the left leg and decreased abdominal reflexes could be detected, which was interpreted as a mild residual of his left hemaparesis. On clinical examination there were no gross deficits in his sensorium and mental status. An EEG made on February 7, 1962, was interpreted as abnormal, representing pathological activity consisting of scattered sharp waves and slightly slower frequency in the right parietal temporal region.

Psychological testing was done on February 21, 1962. His mother, who reported his current difficulties in school, seemed quite anxious about his progress and emphasized her strong wishes for him to go to college. No problems were encountered during psychological testing. His performance on the Wechsler Intelligence Scale for Children (Information, Comprehension, Similarities, Digit Span, Picture Completion, Block Design and Coding Subtest) was somewhat unique. No problems were encountered on an immediate memory task (Digit Span). His performance on this and on most other subtests was well within normal limits (estimated full scale IQ 96). However, he performed very poorly on the coding subtest. The association of numbers and novel symbols was a very difficult task for him. Drawings on the Bender-Gestalt were adequately made and contained no suggestion of visual-perceptual-motor impairment. Human figure drawings were considered to be normal.

It was the impression of the psychologist that this patient's difficulty in school work may be explained more by distractibility and short attention span than by a memory defect *per se*, if such a distinction can be made. His overall intellectual ability was thought to be average, and his present ability in reading was commensurate with his general intelligence. Performance on various tests was thought to be consistent enough generally to preclude any general decrease in intellectual ability as a result of his injury. It was felt possible that if he were capable of better concentration, his school work would improve. There were no obvious emotional complications or overlay. Assurance could not be given to the mother that he would be able to do college work successfully.

It was necessary for him to repeat his grade during the school year 1962-63. On repeat, his work was better although he still had much of the same difficulty. Dexadrine appeared to be of some value in effecting improvement in school work. A repeat EEG on February 26, 1962, indicated a lesser amount of disturbance than the one previous. He was taken off Dilantin without overt difficulty. His school work grades have improved, although he still is not a good student and his school program has been slanted away from a college preparatory course. At the time of his last visit in August 1965, the mother reported that he continued to have some difficulty with memory; study organization was poor; his daily work was fairly good, but he consistently fell down in performance on tests. He showed a great deal of persistence in detailed work such as drafting and did it well. He continued to have to put forth a considerable amount of study in order to perform satisfactorily in his school work. This coming year he has plans to attend a vocational training college in Michigan.

In this case, although objective testing reveals very minimal disturbance, by performance and past hisotry (teachers who previously taught this child felt he was an exceptional student) there has been a definite change in mental ability.

Case 2: S. B., a thirteen-year-old white male, suffered a head injury on August 8, 1963, in an automobile-scooter accident, with loss of consciousness initially and what the mother describes as a semi-comatose state for one week. Neurosurgical evaluation on August 8, 1963, indicated impaired hearing in the left ear, mild left facial weakness and early papilledema. The patient was subsequently operated in Memphis on August 20, 1963, with findings of a small subdural hydroma on the right, and a large extradural hematoma in the left temporal fossa. He was discharged from the hospital on September 5, 1963, following surgery. History from the mother and physicians' reports indicate persistent difficulty with school work during the school years 1963-64 and 1964-65. He was in the seventh and eighth grades at this time and his mother noted (in addition to his difficulty with school work) nervousness, frustration, quick temper, irritable behavior and periodic headaches. The family and teachers reported they noticed particular difficulty with memory. His grades this current year are "B's" in spelling and math, and "D's" in history and English. By report of the family, teacher, and family physician this patient's academic performance prior to his injury was considerably superior to this. Initial skull x-rays prior to surgery indicated a parietal fracture extending into the base, abnormal EEG over the left hemisphere prior to the surgery and a normal EEG in November 1963. Follow-up neurosurgical evaluations indicated a normal neurosurgical exam, with diagnosis of a moderately severe head injury, with the possibility that some of his psychological and adjustment difficulties could be related to the effects of the accident. The ENT examination indicated a 40 to 50 per cent hearing loss in the left ear. The mother also reported some mild difficulty with coordination.

Examination on February 19, 1965, indicated a pleasant cooperative child who had no apparent difficulty with language. On brief mental-status examination, he did not have much difficulty on immediate recall, but manifested considerable difficulty and anxiety in performing serial subtractions; he also made frequent mistakes with perseverative type errors. The neuromuscular examination indicated a mild left facial weakness and asymmetry; mild difficulty in performance of heel-to-knee test; mild difficulty with rapid hopping on the left side as compared to the right; and slight asymmetry on the left-sided abdominal reflexes. EEG examination at this time was thought to be within normal limits.

On psychological examination the patient was cooperative, stating he was aware that he had had some forgetfulness since his accident of August 1963. Testing on the WISC indicated an overall depression of intellectual efficiency with only the subtests of general comprehension being above the average in the verbal tests. The other tests were considerably below the mean, giving the boy an intelligence quotient of 94 with the verbal material. The performance rating was 93. There was felt to be an impairment of concentration and attention rather than actual impairment of general intelligence. Irritability, anxiety, and willingness to accept an inferior response in order to move on was apparent. It was felt this was compatible with the changes seen in postconcussion syndrome, and probably accounted for his marked intellectual inefficiency. On the Kohs Block Design similar type of inefficiency was apparent. The Bender-Gestalt figures showed distortions which suggested some difficulty in perception, with occasional loss in the overall configuration.

The summary opinion was that this boy's performance was consistent with the postconcussion syndrome with general inefficiency of intellectual performance secondary to the injury. It was felt some improvement in control of general affective response would result in more efficient intellectual performance, and that the findings themselves did not exclude anxiety as a cause for his performance on the examination.

Discussion: Both of these patients had (by the definition of Russell and Smith) a severe, to very severe cerebral concussion;

both had surgery for extra-cerebral accumulation of blood, one had a skull fracture and both, at an interval of greater than a year subsequent to the injury, were manifesting significant academic and behavioral disturbance which would not be easily attributable to any cause other than the head injury. In contrast to this, psychological testing by several experienced examiners, neurological examination and EEG reveal minimal or equivocal findings which, to requote Richardson, ". . . in no way represent the long-term crippling effects of the injury on the patient." There has been a tendency in the past to try to separate the affective disturbances of head injury and focus on objective impairment as an indication of organicity. It appears to be true that it is not really possible or meaningful to make this rather artificial distinction.

There may be a tendency to view affective disturbance as a functional effect, since it is so prominent in psychoneurotic reactions, when, in actual fact, it may be one of the prominent residuals of organic dysfunction following head injury. Conversely, as pointed out by Tooth, difficulties with memory adversely affecting test scores is common to psychoneurotic states as well as post-concussion states.

In both cases, the actual day-to-day performance in the home and classroom seems to be a more sensitive index of impairment than anything we can obtain by specific examination. This performance is probably an excellent guide regarding eventual prognosis.

Although the process of memory storage and recall is undoubtedly more complicated than we can presently suppose, the idea of macromolecular protein specification by electrical excitation provides an attractive model. As proposed by Dixon (1962) disturbance in memory after concussion may represent mechanically-induced disorder in an elaborate coding system. Recovery may depend on the ability of glia and nerve cells to restore specific macromolecular configurations. Also, the restoration or compensation for fiber tracts injured or disrupted (as shown by Strich) may require considerable time, and yet be incomplete.

In view of the clinical and laboratory evidence that the

temporal regions of the brain, particularly hippocampus and entero-rhinal cortex, have a crucial function in processing, storage and recall of information, we may speculate that concussion has a particular effect on these structures. This is further suggested by the fact that relatively small lesions, as in Korsakoff's syndrome, may produce a profound disturbance in memory. Since these same areas subserve not only memory, but also facilitation and control of affective responses, it is not perhaps surprising to observe both present in the same patient or to see affect interfere with performance.

REFERENCES

1. DILLON, H., AND LEOPOLD, R. L.: Children and the post concussion syndrome. *JAMA, 175*:86, 1961.
2. DIXON, K. C.: The amnesia of cerebral concussion. *Lancet, ii*:1359, 1962.
3. MAGOUN, H. W.: The Waking Brain, 2nd ed. Springfield, Thomas, 1963, chap. 8.
4. OLDFIELD, R. C., AND WILLIAMS, M.: *J Neurol Neurosurg Psychiat, 24*:32, 1961.
5. RICHARDSON, F.: Some effects of severe head injury. *Develop Med Child Neurol, 5*:471, 1963.
6. ROWBOTHAM, G. F., *et al.*: Analysis of 1,400 cases of acute injury to the head. *Brit Med J, 1*:726, 1954.
7. RUSSELL, W. R.: Cerebral involvement in head injury. *Brain, 55*:549, 1932.
8. RUSSELL, W. R., AND SMITH, A.: Post-traumatic amnesia in closed head injury. *Arch Neurol, 5*:4, 1961.
9. SILVERMAN: EEG study of acute head injury in children. *Neurology, 12*:273, 1962.
10. STRICH, S. J.: Diffuse degeneration of the cerebral white matter in severe dementia following head injury. *J Neurol Psychiat, 19*:163, 1956.
11. STRICH, S. J., Shearing of nerve fibers as a cause of brain damage due to head injury. *Lancet, ii*:443, 1961.
12. TOOTH, G.: On the use of mental tests for the measurement of disability after head injury. *J Neurol Psychiat, 10*:1, 1947.
13. WATSON, J. D., AND CRICK, F. H.: Genetic implications of the structure of DNA. *Nature, 171*:964, 1953.

IX

INDICATIONS FOR PSYCHOLOGICAL EVALUATION IN MENTAL RETARDATION AND NEUROLOGICAL DISORDERS

J. T. JABBOUR, M.D.

THE NEED for psychological evaluation of children has often been determined by parents, teachers, physicians, or social workers. This evaluation, like the pediatric, neurological, or any other laboratory examination, was requested because of a "slow child," a child with a learning problem; more recently, because of the child with behavior problems, a convulsive disorder, or "minimal cerebral dysfunction" (1, 2, 3, 4, 5).

In some patients, an abnormal EEG or a school report card has led to such an evaluation. Recently, recognition of preventable disorders, i.e., premature infants; remedial disorders (phenylketonuric infants); or often treatable conditions, i.e. convulsive disorders or hyperactive behavioral syndromes have challenged physicians to utilize not only clinical and laboratory studies, but also psychological evaluation in order to aid in planning and management of the patient and his family. Several features of these neurological disorders, from the very obvious to those very subtle abnormalities which contribute to recognition of the problem, are described as more experience is gained in these children who have mental, learning, and behavioral problems.

FEATURES OBSERVED IN NEUROLOGICAL DISORDERS

Face

The appearance of slanted eyes; flat bridge of the nose; epicanthic folds; enlarged tongue in an elliptical shaped mouth;

194

or other body stigmata, announce Down's syndrome, even to the observant parent or medical student. On the other hand, the features of the first arch syndrome are less obvious even to the experienced physician, although this syndrome has been known for some time and was recently reviewed by McKenzie (6). The features of micrognathia, hypertelorism, ear anomalies, mandibulofacial dysostosis, and cleft lip and palate are not fully appreciated by most physicians. Many patients with such features have mental and/or language retardation, or a convulsive disorder. The facial features may also appear in parents or siblings of these children. The pathogenesis is probably related to both a strong genetic and environmental influence on the stapedial artery, which does not maintain its blood supply to facial structures.

Other disorders with facial features include the deLange syndrome with a small nose, micrognathia, eyebrows growing together, thin lips with a downward curve and an expressionless face (7). The oral-facial-digital syndrome of hypertelorism or hypotelorism: small alar cartilages, a median cleft like defect of the upper lip, a lobulated bifid or multifid tongue with digital abnormalities of syndactyly or polydactyly, may indicate mental retardation. This syndrome has a dominant inheritance occurring only in females and is lethal to the male (8).

The growth and shape of the head is usually dependent on brain growth, maturation and development. The usual measurement of the occipital frontal circumference is well-known, but rarely equated with the rapidity of brain and infant development. The head may grow more than one centimeter each month during the first year of life; by four years of age, over 80 per cent of the head circumference is achieved. The brain in a normal newborn is 335 grams at birth and by one year of age weighs 900 grams, or two pounds. This growth and development not only of the brain, but also of the child, is dependent on the normal electrophysiological and neurochemical maturation (9).

Within the first eighteen months of life, the presence of either microcephaly and macrocephaly (either primary or developmental in origin) may be evident. Too often, the head circumference is not correlated with the mental ability; however, renewed interest in the head circumference and mental ability has recently been studied. In a series of 134 children with a head circumference below two standard deviations or more, all children had mental subnormality except one (10).

Macrocephaly of either heredofamilial origin, or related to syndromes such as Hurler's disease, achrondoplasia; or other progressive neurological disorders, such as hydrocephalus or cerebral lipidosis may also be observed.

Body

The tall or short body may indicate such disorders as deLange or Down's syndrome, or the connective tissue disorders such as Hurler's or Marfan's disease, all associated with mental retardation (11). Facial, cranial, skeletal or cardiovascular defects aid in the diagnosis of these disorders.

Muscle

Hemiatrophy and hemihypertrophy may be associated with cerebral dysfunction. Spastic hemiplegia occurs more often than any other type of cerebral palsy, and usually may result from damage to the frontal, parietal, or temporal lobe. Hemihypertrophy is considered to be a form of the neurocutaneous syndromes in which there is a diffuse abnormality resulting in mental or behavioral alteration (12).

Skin

The neurocutaneous syndromes, Sturge-Weber disease, tuberous sclerosis and neurofibromatosis have characteristic skin lesions. These disorders have a variable hereditary pattern, and form frustes which are frequently observed in children with psychological and mental alteration. The cause of mental retardation and convulsions in these disorders is not known (13, 14).

Sturge-Weber disease consists of hemiconvulsions, hemiatrophy, the port wine hemangioma of the face, and mental retardation. There is usually typical linear skull calcification.

Tuberous sclerosis consists of angioma, fibroma or adenoma

sebaceum of the face, generalized or focal convulsions and mental retardation. Other systemic components permit diagnosis without difficulty. In many patients, *cafe-au-lait* skin lesions, hemangioma, shagreen skin or subungal fibroma of the fingernails are observed.

Neurofibromatosis is the most common of the neurocutaneous syndromes. Although many patients may develop neurofibromas; meningiomas or gliomas along the spinal cord; roots, or brain structures, many patients with only a few *cafe-au-lait* skin lesions and a family history of a neurocutaneous disorder, may have either mental retardation, behavioral or convulsive disorder. Thus, such obvious and unusual features may herald the presence of a cerebral dysfunction requiring psychological evaluation.

DISORDERS OF CEREBRAL DYSFUNCTION

Neurophysiological Studies

These disorders are at best related to neurophysiological disturbances previously studied in both animal and man, and may be appropriately reviewed before these entities are described.

There is voluminous literature (on the role of various areas of the brain) which may contribute to behavior and learning. These are of a complex nature, and the most striking findings have been observed in either ablation or stimulation of certain areas of the brain. The well-known study of Kluver and Bucy of bilateral temporal lobectomy produced striking alterations in monkeys such as fearlessness, tameness, docility and emotional unresponsiveness which were thought to be caused by the ablation of the amygdala and pyriform lobe (15). In contrast, stimulation of the amygdala induced fear and rage, while focal lesions of the amygdala or pyriform cortex produced docility and hypersexuality in animals (16).

In recent years, unilateral and bilateral amygdalectomy in sixty patients ranging from five to thirty-five years of age was performed by stereotaxic oil wax destruction of the amygdala in an effort to modify behavior (17). Forty-six of these patients had generalized and/or psychomotor convulsions. In fifty-one of the patients, this procedure resulted in marked reduction in emotional excitability and normalization of the patient's social behavior and adaptation. Progress of such studies from animal to man are slow, but certainly add to both our understanding of the disorder and to the possible modes of therapy.

In both man and animal, a loss of aggression follows amygdalectomy because of reduced facilitory influence on lower mechanisms altering aggressive behavior. Hyperphagia and hypersexuality both suggest that the amygdala has an inhibitory influence on the lower mechanisms for both alimentary and sexual behavior (16, 18).

In patients with temporal lobe seizures, temporal lobe stimulation results in actual earlier remembered experience. It is believed that the hippocampus and the adjacent entorhinal temporal cortex induce, as well as consolidate, memory and early recall. The ascending reticular influences upon the cerebral hemispheres are concerned with initiating and modifying arousal, wakefulness, orienting, and attention (8). Locomotor hyperactivity occurs after frontal cortical ablation of orbital frontal area 13, and is believed to be caused by the removal of inhibition upon neural pathways serving motility (19). These studies suggest that many areas of the brain may be involved in those individuals who have modified mental, learning, and psychological behavior. It would seem from studies of children with mental retardation and brain damage, that isolated lobes or areas of the brain are rarely involved, but that altered pathways serving several structures result in these clinical disorders (Figure 1).

Minimal Brain Dysfunction

Recently, the term for minimal brain dysfunction, "subtle cerebral palsy," has plagued physicians, educators and psychologists (Table I). This syndrome consists of behavioral, learning and motor problems or convulsive disorders. The convulsive disorders and hyperactive behavior problems may not

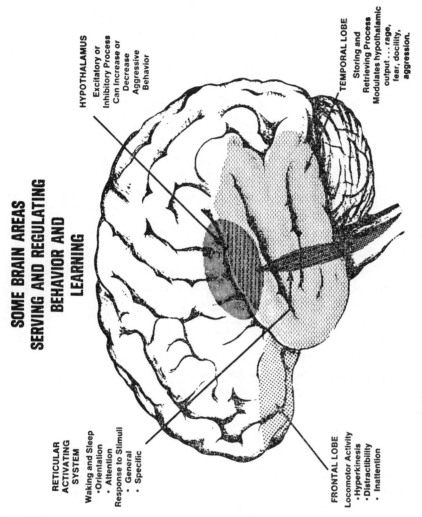

SOME BRAIN AREAS SERVING AND REGULATING BEHAVIOR AND LEARNING

HYPOTHALAMUS
Excitatory or Inhibitory Process Can Increase or Decrease Aggressive Behavior

TEMPORAL LOBE
Storing and Retrieving Process Modulates hypothalamic output . . . rage, fear, docility, aggression.

RETICULAR ACTIVATING SYSTEM
Waking and Sleep
•Orientation
• Attention
Response to Stimuli
• General
• Specific

FRONTAL LOBE
Locomotor Activity
•Hyperkinesis
•Distractibility
• Inattention

be fully appreciated by physicians and educators; while the confirmation of motor and learning problems are easily demonstrated by detailed examination searching for movement or motor abnormalities, perceptual or conceptual problems.

The causal factors are often poorly documented, variable in both time and effect on the child. They may be related only in that the causal factor triggers a latent defect such as the convulsive threshold; circumstances permit the disturbance to appear either gradually or suddenly. If carefully interrogated,

TABLE I
MINIMAL CEREBRAL DYSFUNCTION
EPILEPSY
Psychomotor
Convulsive Equivalent
BEHAVIOR PROBLEMS
Hyperactive
Erratic
Unpredictable
MOTOR DYSFUNCTION
Clumsy Child
Choreiform Syndrome
LEARNING DISABILITY
Percept
Concept
Language

the patient with the disorder may have had it from early infancy.

The age of onset is variable and the features in these disorders may overlap. The clinical correlation with EEG and neuroanatomical findings may provide a better understanding of the spectrum of disturbances and how it can best be recognized as a diagnostic entity.

Convulsive Disorders

Children with convulsive disorders have sudden, recurrent episodes, or attacks of either motor, sensory, psychic, or visceral alteration of either a generalized or focal nature. The generalized *grand mal* convulsion, with typical features of tonus and/or clonus with unconsciousness and postictal sleep, is easily recognized. The absence or lapse of *petit mal* may be overlooked, but is readily confirmed by the recording of the three-per-second spike and wave pattern. Similarly, the myoclonic seizure in the infant, or the akinetic seizure in the older child have classic EEG patterns. Focal motor convulsions, adversive, Jacksonian march, or postural seizures may be confirmed by the EEG localization to the frontal lobe. These convulsive disorders may have accompanying psychological, behavioral or mental disturbances, including mental retardation, which rarely go unrecognized by either the parent, teacher, or physician.

Convulsive Equivalent and Psychomotor Convulsions

Two similar disorders, differing only in clinical and EEG features, are frequently observed (Table II). Children with

TABLE II

COMPARATIVE FEATURES OF PSYCHOMOTOR CONVULSIONS
AND CONVULSIVE EQUIVALENT

	PSYCHOMOTOR CONVULSIONS	CONVULSIVE EQUIVALENTS
INCIDENCE	15-30%	10%
ETIOLOGY		
HEREDOFAMILIAL	20-30%	20-30%
AGE YEARS	3-6	6-9
ASSOCIATED PROBLEMS		
RETARDATION	20%.	30%
BEHAVIOR	20%	40%
LEARNING PERCEPTUAL	15%	20%
EEG PATTERN		
MEDICATION RESPONSE	85%	85%
BEHAVIOR	Improved Worsened	Improved No Effect
SEIZURE	HEADACHE	HEADACHE
	ABDOMINAL DISCOMFORT	ABDOMINAL PAIN
	STARING	PALLOR, FLUSHING, CYANOSIS
	FUGUE	NAUSEA, VOMITING
	AUTOMATISM	DIZZINESS
	LIP SMACKING - CHEWING	
	VERTIGO, TINNITUS	
	FEAR	
	POSTICTAL SLEEP	
	AMNESIA	

convulsive equivalent and psychomotor convulsions have psychological, behavioral, motor, speech disorders and mental retardation. The convulsive equivalent represents a controversial entity in the pediatric, neurological, and psychological literature. Once prevalent among physicians, the failure to recognize and appreciate psychomotor seizures has now been rectified; thus, we can expect greater numbers of both disorders with time and experience (3, 4).

The paroxysmal nature of the attack; the causal and hereditary factors; the associated problems of behavior, learning and mental retardation, exist in both. These entities differ only in the features of the attack, the EEG patterns, the age of onset and the response to medication. This is best illustrated in the table.

Hyperactive behavior syndrome (a complex of annoying signs and symptoms) is highly indicative of cerebral dysfunction and can best be related to frontal temporal lobe damage and/or dysfunction. Features include hyperactivity; impulsivity; emotional lability; short attention span; distractibility; variable performance; low frustration tolerance; perseveration, and specific learning defects (2, 20). These are frequently associated with neurological and electroencephalographic abnormality. Recent studies of 780 patients by electroencephalographic study demonstrate abnormality in 60 per cent of children with a hyperactive behavior syndrome alone; up to 90 per cent of children if the hyperactive syndrome accompanies other neurological abnormalities (19). The results of the neurological examination may be similar to that described in children with convulsive equivalent, psychomotor convulsive disorder, or minimal cerebral dysfunction.

Children with these disorders not only have variable signs and symptoms, but also exhibit variable physical and neurological findings often designated as "soft," "minimal," "transient," or equivocal in contrast to "persistent" or definite neurological signs. It is from this feature that the term "minimal" is derived, but "minimal" does not mean these problems are of little concern to parents, the child, psychologist or physician. Thus, the differentiation and designation of these problems, which require psychological evaluation, challenge all to search for several areas of disturbed function. The designation of a convulsive, learning, behavior syndrome seems workable. It also provides a more complete look at the problem and a broader approach to the management of the child and his family (Table III). The psychologist is challenged by the learning and emotional disturbances, while the physician must become knowledgeable in the convulsive, behavior and motor disorders; the physician must

TABLE III

CEREBRAL DYSFUNCTION SYNDROME
OR
CONVULSIVE, LEARNING AND BEHAVIOR SYNDROME

Syndrome	Convulsion	Learning	Behavior	Motor	Emotional Disturbance
Hyperactive Behavior	1	1	2	1	1
Convulsive Equivalent	1	2	2	1	1
Psychomotor Epilepsy	2	1	1	0	1

Key: 0 – absent   1 – subtle   2 – apparent

think in terms of management of the total problem—not of a specific problem. For example, the control of convulsions or behavior alone may be accomplished by medication, while academic achievement and emotional disturbances are overlooked.

If the abnormal signs and symptoms are searched for and graded, one may clarify this dynamic and changing neurological disorder, and thus be aware of the complexities of the problem. A score of 0-2 may grade the absence or presence of a subtle or apparent disorder. The higher the score, perhaps, the more complex the problem. Even with this grading, however, a problem in one area still requires careful evaluation and management. These are not *minimal disorders* for the child, physician, psychologist, or the parents. This is adequately shown by both the number and problems in both diagnosis and management.

REFERENCES

1a. CLEMENTS, S. D., AND PETERS, J. E.: Minimal brain dysfunctions in the schoolage child. *Arch Gen Psychol*, 6:185-197, 1962.

1b. MacKEITH, R., AND BAX, M. (Ed.): Minimal cerebral dysfunction. Little Club Clinics in *Develop Med Child Neurol, 10,* 1963.

2. LAUFER, M. W., AND DENHOFF, E.: Hyperkinetic behavior syndrome in children. *J Pediat, 50*:463-474, 1957.

3. CHAO, D., SEXTON, J. A., AND DAVIS, S. D.: Convulsive equivalent syndrome of childhood. *J Pediat, 64*:499-508, 1964.

4. CHAO, D., SEXTON, J. A., AND PARDO, L. S. S.: Temporal lobe epilepsy in children. *J Pediat, 60*:686-693, 1962.

5. WILSON, W. P., AND HARRIS, B. S. H.: Psychiatric problems in children with frontal, central, and temporal lobe epilepsy. *Southern Med J,* 59:49-52, 1966.

6. McKenzie, J.: First arch syndrome. *Arch Dis Child, 33*:477-486, 1958.
7. Ptacek, L. J., Opitz, J. M., Smith, D. W., Gerritsen, T., and Waisman, H. A.: Cornelia deLange syndrome. *J Pediat, 63*:1000-1020, 1963.
8. Ruess, A. L., Pruzansky, S., Lis, E. F., and Patau, K.: Oral-facial digital syndrome: A multiple congenital condition of females with associated chromosomal abnormalities. *Pediatrics, 29*:95-995, 1962.
9. Dekaban, A.: *Neurology of Infancy.* Baltimore, Williams & Wilkins, 1959.
10. O'Connell, E. J., Feldt, R. H., and Stickler, G. B.: Head circumference, mental retardation, growth failure. *Pediatrics, 36*:62-66, 1965.
11. McKusick, V. A.: *Heritable Disorders of Connective Tissue.* St. Louis, Mosby, 1956.
12. Ringrose, R. E., Jabbour, J. T., and Keele, D. K.: Hemihypertrophy. *Pediatrics, 36*:434, 1965.
13. Merritt, H. H.: *Textbook of Neurology.* Philadelphia, Lea and Febiger, 1963.
14. Canale, D., Bebin, J., and Knighton, R. S.: Neurologic manifestations of Von Recklinghausen's disease of the nervous system. *Confin Neurol, 24*:359-403, 1964.
15. Kluver, H., and Buch, P. C.: Preliminary analysis of functions of the temporal lobes in monkeys. *Arch Neurol Psychiat, 42*:979-1000, 1939.
16. Ursin, H., and Kaada, B. R.: Functional localization within the amygdaloid complex in the cat. *Electroenceph Clin Neurophysiol, 12*:1-20, 1960.
17. Narabayshi, H., et al.: Stereotaxic amygdaletomy for behavior disorders. *Arch Neurol, 9*:1-16, 1963.
18. Magoun, H. W.: *The Waking Brain.* Springfield, Thomas, 1963.
19. Ruch, T. C., and Shenkin, H. A.: The relation of area 13 on orbital surface of frontal lobes to hyperactivity and hyperphagia in monkeys. *J Neurophysiol, 6*:349-360, 1943.
20. Klinkerfuss, G. H., Lange, P. H., Wienberg, W. A., and O'Leary, J. D.: Electroencephalographic abnormalities of children with hyperkinetic behavior. *Neurology, 15*:883-891.

DISCUSSION I

T. S. Hill, M.D.

The presentations of Dr. Mackey on "Problems in Evaluation of Residual Effects of Head Injury" and Dr. Jabbour clearly demonstrate that the "Indications for Psychological Evaluation in Mental Retardation and Neurological Disorders" (to make use of Dr. Jabbour's subject) may be several in number and varied in nature.

Their examples of neurological disorders include those which began before, during, and after birth. Thus, there were those of genetic (hereditary) origin, as in heredo-familial conditions cited, and those of congenital origin. Others had their inception during the neonatal or, actually, during the natal period, with the head injuries having been incurred postnatally.

The physician who possesses a knowledge of the significance of these groupings of anatomical and functional abnormalities (and so far as is known, their etiology) endeavors to search for evidence of associated mental, emotional, or behavioral aberrations. This he does first through a history obtained from parents, teachers and others; next, by carefully performed interview, physical and neurological examinations, as well as laboratory studies. By these studies he may, in some patients, readily find evidence of deficit in the patient's behavior, emotional reactions, or intelligence. He may also see that dysfunction in any one or more of these areas affects progress in learning. However, as in some of the conditions described in these papers, he may encounter difficulty in detecting any abnormalities in these spheres, although he may suspect them to be present, at least to a minor degree. Hence, in some instances, the most important indication for a skilled psychological evaulation may be to ascertain the existence or nonexistence of mental retardation or personality change. But whenever dysfunction is detected, it is imperative to obtain as accurate a delineation as possible of the nature and extent thereof. Here, a carefully chosen battery of psychological tests best serves this purpose. Failure to utilize them deprives the physician of information essential for the most comprehensive and beneficial method of treatment and handling.

Whereas the referring physician should have a reasonably adequate comprehension of the various types and nature of both objective and projective tests and information they may provide, rarely does his own training qualify him to select, administer, or make detailed interpretations of such tests. The physician must seek the aid of the well-trained psychologist to perform these functions. Such remarks made in our academic center seem so elemental; yet years of observation show that their emphasis is still required.

As Dr. Jabbour has indicated, referrals may come from many sources whenever the history warrants a request for psychological evaluation. One wonders how often, in settings outside of special clinics, it is the request of a parent (made, perhaps, at the urging of a teacher, or a social worker, rather than at the initial appraisal and decision of the physician) which generates the referral for psychological evaluation.

Some of the inquiries being made at this institute attest to the present day need for improvement in the construction and interpretation of certain psychological tests needed to demonstrate more sensitively any evidence of organic brain change. The same may hold for many other tests, such as those for certain aspects of behavior and attitudes. There could also be improvement of tests for the intellectual, the affective, and other aspects of personality, as well as the sociometric, stress, frustration and vocational aptitude tests. Despite such short-coming, the value now accredited to psychological testing establishes it as a most important supplementary method of study, not only in the types of neurological conditions which have been presented, but also in the whole area of child development which has gained emphasis in the field of pediatrics. One ventures to predict that in either the full-time or attending staff roster of many a university department of pediatrics, there will be included in the future not only the pediatric neurologist, but also the clinical psychologist, the pediatric social worker, and the child psychiatrist. The clinical conditions presented in these papers indicate that for a truly comprehensive psychological evaluation, such an interdisciplinary approach is needed.

Is it possible (not only in brain-damaged patients but in any patient) to interpret accurately some of the measures used to determine the ability for abstract or concrete conceptualizations without a good knowledge of the social-psychological milieu in which he moves? The information to provide this is most competently gathered and interpreted by the trained social worker. Parenthetically, it would be of interest to know whether the benefits derived from Operation Head Start of the Economic Opportunity Act will include any improved rating on intelligence tests, as compared with ratings made on children with equivalent social backgrounds who had not been in the program. It would seem to be of greatest importance that the approach to a psychological evaluation in a medical setting be holistic in nature. In such an approach, utilization of psychological tests is but one aspect of a total psychological evaluation.

So often during a psychological evaluation, the engrossment in detecting the existence or nonexistence of deficits, the assessment of their nature and extent is so great, that the most important parameter of all may be overlooked or given scant attention. The degree and nature of the defect in a brain-damaged child may be intensively studied, but how complete an examination is made of the quantity, quality, and usability of his remaining resources? On the basis of intelligence measurement, one child is declared trainable whereas another is designated to be educable, but how complete is the appraisal of the child's special interests and aptitudes? How much effort is really expended in determining the nature, reason for, and treatability of the expressed emotional and behavioral patterns which can seriously limit full use of his intelligence?

Is there a tendency to make less extensive the battery of tests applied to determine a child's full potentialities, once evidence of brain damage has been obtained, even though this may be minimal in extent? The challenge is great to obtain a most complete evaluation during educational and vocational guidance of the youth with superior intelligence. Should it be less with the brain-damaged child? Are not the erratic, explosive episodes of behavior attributed solely to a loss of control due to brain damage? How carefully is the history taken, the interview made and the testing done, to reveal the degree of conflict and existence of neurotic mechanisms which may more realistically account for a part of this behavior? In evaluating the effects of cerebral pathology upon any individual, it should be remembered that as Brosin (1959) has stated, they operate upon ". . . a living human being 'who is a part of all he has met' and has flexible identity only in terms of the social-psychological matrix in which he moves."

The difficulties in diagnosis and understanding of the child with minimal brain damage have been stressed by Dr. Mackey and Dr. Jabbour. These serve to remind us it is equally important to be certain that brain damage as a causal factor in many of the behavior and learning disorders is excluded. All too often it is not.

REFERENCES

BROSIN, HENRY W.: Psychiatric conditions following head injury. In *American Handbook of Psychiatry*. New York, Basic Books, 1959.

DISCUSSION II

F. S. HILL, M.D.

This speaker will present case reports. They will tend to give practical clinical substance to the theoretical considerations already heard.

CASE 1.: J. C. was the product of an uncomplicated pregnancy, labor and delivery. His development was normal during early infancy. He sat alone at six months and crawled at seven months of age. When the patient was eight and one-half months old, he suffered bilateral, parietal-temporal, subdural hematomas as a result of an automobile accident. Three craniotomies were performed over the next three month period. Subsequent to these events, J. C. again had to learn to sit alone and to crawl. However, he did learn to walk at 16 months, and it was the opinion of his mother that his speech was delayed by three-to-four months. During the next five years, the patient was treated for the usual childhood diseases, requiring repeated physical examinations. No gross neurological abnormalities were observed. However, a general "immaturity" was noted during the office visits.

The child entered kindergarten at age five, but it was felt by his teacher that his progress was not sufficient for entrance into the first grade. When he was five years and eleven months old psychological evaluation was performed. The following results were obtained as listed below:

1. The examiner was impressed by his immaturity.
2. His speech was that of a three and one-half to four year old child.

3. He possessed an extremely brief attention span.
4. His Stanford-Binet intelligence quotient was estimated at 92.
5. His Human Figure Drawing intelligence was estimated at 90.
6. His intelligence was low normal on both reading readiness and number readiness on the Metropolitan readiness tests.
7. He had an inability to follow directions.
8. Perseveration was noticed.
9. He possessed an inability to do simplest block designs.
10. He produced fragmented drawings particularly on the Bender-Gestalt Test.
11. He gave twenty-one responses on the Rorschach but fixed on the phrase "torn up" on almost all the percepts and reeled them off in a mechanical staccato fashion.
12. The examiner felt that in addition to the probable organic involvement, overprotectiveness and sheltering by the parents augmented the difficulties.

The electroencephalographic patterns were normal in both sleeping and waking states.

At the present time, this patient is repeating kindergarten. His mother feels definite progress has been made. He will be placed in a special class for perceptually handicapped children at the beginning of the next school term. An interesting sidelight is that his present teacher has stated he could do better if he weren't lazy.

This case report illustrates the diffuse, nonspecific intellectual deficit which may be produced by brain injury in infancy.

CASE 2: This report is presented in the interest of early case-finding of patients with minimal brain dysfunction, and is an example of Hyperactive Behavior Syndrome.

Bill, age three years, has been a patient since birth. Growth and development were normal. When he was two years and ten months old, Bill's mother asked for a consultation concerning his behavior. Throughout most of the hour's interview she fought to hold back tears, at times being unable to do so. Her complaint was that her home was kept in shambles by the hyperactivity of this child whom she was unable to control. Bill also showed emotional lability manifest by such things as crying while watching television. The past history revealed the following:

1. Because of previous miscarriage due to incompetent cervix, ligation of the internal cervical os had been performed after pregnancy was well established.
2. Labor lasted about two and one-half hours. The ligation material had stretched and vaginal delivery was done rather than the planned delivery by cesarean section.

3. The immediate newborn period lasted without complication.

4. Colic was present for six months.

5. The mother stated that during infancy the patient never seemed to enjoy cuddling. She said that she often thought, "If he would only let me cuddle him."

Although great difficulty was experienced in obtaining a sleep record, the electroencephalogram was reported to be normal.

The patient was given Chlorpromazine, the dose being ten milligrams three times a day. The mother states he now seems to be a different child. On one occasion she failed to refill the prescription, but stated that after three days she could not get to the pharmacy fast enough. This case also has an interesting sidelight in that the father had attempted to control the child's behavior with the belt.

The present plan for this patient is to maintain control of his hyperactivity with medication. At a later time, complete psychological evaluation will be done in order to determine the possible presence of perceptual handicap or specific learning disorder. Special attention will be given to academic achievement, and to the more subtle behavior disorders such as impulsivity, short attention span, distractibility, variable performance, low frustration tolerance and perseveration. Early diagnosis and treatment, leading to parental acceptance of the child's problem, undoubtedly will prevent much of the emotional overlay which so frequently attends delayed diagnosis of minimal brain dysfunction.

AUTHORS CITED

A

Aita, J. A., 52, 56, 84
Altman, J., 121, 127
Aristotle, 110
Armitage, S. G., 66, 84

B

Babcock, H., 56, 84
Baer, D. M., 37, 38
Barclay, A., 29, 103, 104
Barrett, B. H., 35, 36, 37, 38
Bauman, M. K., 149
Baumeister, A., 108
Bax, M., 194, 202, 203
Bayley, N., 117, 128
Beadle, G. W., 112, 115
Bebin, J., 196, 204
Becker, 97
Belmont, L., 23, 38
Bender, L., 50, 84
Bensberg, G. J., 146, 149
Berman, P. W., 27, 34, 38
Beverly, L., 146, 149
Bijou, S. W., 37, 38, 100, 104, 174,
  175
Birch, H. G., 23, 25, 26, 38,
  105-106, 108
Birch, J. R., 140, 146, 149-150
Birch, J. W., 140, 146, 149-150
Birnbrauer, J. S., 37, 38
Blodgett, H. E., 156, 175
Boone, J. N., 140
Braine, Martin, 119, 128
Brosin, H. W., 207, 208
Brown, D. W., 140, 145, 148, 150
Bucy, P. C., 197, 205
Burke, B. S., 117, 128
Burke, C. J., 53, 58, 86

C

Canale, D., 196, 204
Canter, A. H., 54, 84
Carroll, L., 180
Castle, P. W., 121, 131
Chao, D., 194, 201, 203
Chow, Bacon, F., 128
Clements, S. D., 194, 203
Comte, A., 41, 43
Cooper, 157
Corah, N. L., 119, 128
Cowley, J. J., 115, 128
Craft, M., 101, 102, 105
Cravioto, J., 119, 128
Crick, F. H., 187, 193
Cromwell, R. L., 108

D

Dabrowski, 166
Darwin, C., 111, 113
Davis, S. D., 194, 201, 203
Deanin, G. G., 116, 128
de Graaf, R., 110
De Grange, M. Q., 41, 43
Dekaban, A., 195, 204
De Licardie, E. R., 119, 128
Delprato, D. J., 91, 93
Denhoff, E., 194, 203
De Vries, H., 111, 113
Diller, L., 25, 26, 38
Dillon, H., 187, 193
Dixon, K. C., 192, 193
Dobbing, J., 128
Doehring, D. G., 64, 84
Doll, E., 18, 19
Dreger, R. M., 146, 150
Dunphy, E. B., 120, 128

211

SUBJECT INDEX

A

AAMD, *see* American Association on Mental Deficiency
Achievement, deprivation's effect, 122
Acquired characteristics, inheritance theory, 111
Adaptation to deficiencies, importance, 11
Adaptive behavior
anatomic, physiologic characteristics and, 25-27
cultural deprivation and, 18
impairment, 6
personality-environment formula, 42
retardation factor, 5
technology and, 16
Adults
retarded, differences from children, 20, 23-24
Affective deficits
mental retardation and, 99-100
Aged, *see* Geriatric center and Geriatric services
Alcoholism
socioeconomic factors, 5
American Association on Mental Deficiency
Classification Manual, updating importance, 13
definition of mental retardation, 5-6
comprehensive center's role, 10-11
Amnesia
post-traumatic, 186-187
Animal studies
deprivation's effects, 126, 127
malnutrition's effects, 115, 116-117
stimulation's effects, 121
Aphasia
case report, 173
tests for, 58-59, 66, 71

Auditory skills
assessment importance, 11
Autistic child
in institution for mentally retarded, 92

B

Behavior
malnutrition's effect, 115, 116
nutrition's effect on, 118, 120, 122
see also Adaptive behavior
Behavioral center
need for, 12
Bender-Gestalt performance
deprivation relationship, 125
Black children, *see* Children, black
Blind children
abilities, 149
function in society, 151-153
individual differences, 152-153
intelligence quotients, 143-145
testing, 148-149
Body
stigmata of neurological disorders, 196
Brain
amygdalectomy, effects, 197-198
areas regulating behavior and learning, 197-199
concussion, classification, 186
development
fetal conditions relationship, 119
nutrition's effect, 120
drugs' effect on, 117
dysfunction, minimal, 198-200
infection's effect, 117
malnutrition's effect on, 117
poverty's effect, 110-131
stimulation needs, 127

psychological evaluation, indications
for, 194-210
"Mikado" (Gilbert and Sullivan), 95
Minority groups
errors in labelling, 8
needs, 127
test results, 123
See also Children, black
Mothers
diet's effect on unborn, 119,
diseases' effect on unborn, 120
influence on unborn, 112-114, 115,
116, 117
nutrition's effect on unborn and
infants, 117, 120, 125
smoking, effect on unborn, 119
See also Fathers, and Parents
Mothers' clubs
professional help in, 174
Motivation
deprivation's effect, 126
test result relationship, 125
Motor skills
assessment important, 11
socioeconomic leevl relationship, 123
Mumps' effect on unborn, 120
Muscles
changes due to neurological
disorders, 196
Mutation
De Vries studies, 111

N

Narcotic addiction
socioeconomic factors, 5
National Association for Brain Injured
aid to parents, 174
National Institute of Neurological
Diseases; *See* Collaborative
Project
Natural selection
Darwin theory, 111
Negro children; *See* Children, black
Neurofibromatosis
external signs, 197
Neurological center
need for, 12

Neurological deficit
deprivation relationship, 122-126
Neurological factors
importance in therapy, 12
See also Brain damage
Neuronal damage due to infectious
diseases, 120
Neuropsychology Laboratory, Indiana
University
analyses of test scores, 58-59
case reports from, 73-84
test battery, 65-73
See also Tests
Nobel Prize, Medicine, 112
Numbers
mentally retarded, 4
Nurses, *See* Public health nurses
Nutrition
deficiency's effects, 121-122
on infants, 119-120
effects on
achievement, 125
behavior, 118, 120
growth, 118
learning ability, 120
mental development, 118
school success, 119
importance, 127
mothers, effect on infants, 117

O

Obstetrical care
importance, 127
Occupational therapy
needs in Down's syndrome, 10
Offices of Education, Vocational
Rehabilitation
development of job families for
handicapped, 151
Onondaga Study, 4, 6
Operation Head Start
programs, 7
Organicity
distinction from brain damage, 41-42
Rorschach signs, 25
signs, 24